**PREC**

Charlotte Clark-Neitzel, M.D.
403 C  Black Hills Lane S.W.
Olympia, WA.  98502

# **PRE**CONCEPTION

*A Woman's Guide to*

*Preparing for*

*Pregnancy and Parenthood*

## **Brenda Aikey-Keller**

John Muir Publications
Santa Fe, New Mexico

*Dedication*

*To my sons, Thomas, Daniel, and Aaron.*
*Without whom I would not have experienced the*
*true joys of life, pregnancy, and parenthood.*

John Muir Publications, P.O. Box 613, Santa Fe, NM 87504

First edition. First printing

LIBRARY OF CONGRESS CATALOGING-IN-PUBLICATION DATA
Aikey-Keller, Brenda, 1957-
  Preconception: a woman's guide to preparing for pregnancy and parenthood/Brenda
Aikey-Keller. — lst ed.
    p. cm.
  Includes bibliographical references.
  ISBN 0-945465-44-0
  1. Pregnancy—Decision making. 2. Pregnant women—Health and hygiene. 3.
Pregnancy—Economic aspects. 4. Parenthood.
I. Title.
RG525.A25   1990
618.2'4—dc20                                                                89-42946
                                                                                 CIP

DISTRIBUTED TO THE TRADE BY:

W. W. Norton & Company, Inc.
New York, New York

Cover illustration: Sally Blakemore
Typographer: Copygraphics, Inc.
Printer: McNaughton & Gunn

# CONTENTS

# PREFACE

This book is about creating the ideal situation into which to bring a child. It is not meant to discourage anyone from having a child but rather to encourage them to make those changes and choices that will allow for a more stable beginning.

The men and women mentioned in this book are real, with different names. They are couples and single women who want to do the best for their children-yet-to-be. They are struggling with their own sense of responsibility as well as with the social standards that are being pushed on them.

Those considering pregnancy owe it to themselves and to their child to prepare the best they can. Like any other aspect of life, when we do not possess control, we can get frustrated and angry. By bringing a child into this world without preparation, couples may feel as if they are losing control of part of their lives.

As a mother, I know what it is not to have prepared. As a woman who has experienced pregnancy, I see now that I had a multitude of choices available to me which I was not assertive enough to choose. As men and women, we deserve to have choices and the privilege to make changes that will enhance our lives and those lives we intend to create.

I would like to thank those friends who have encouraged me and believed in the potential of this book.

I would like to thank George Sheldon, my mentor, my friend, and my coach.

I appreciate all the support I received from my fellow writers; you know who you are.

I thank the women in my life, Sandy, Ruth, Kay, Karen, and Nina, who understand the need for women to make changes and choices for more fulfilling lives.

Jim, I will always appreciate your support and understanding in my need to be creative.

A special thanks to all the couples who allowed me to be part of their prenatal lives. Your experiences and willingness to share have taught me more than you will ever know.

# CHAPTER 1

# BEING PREPARED IS NOT JUST FOR BOY SCOUTS

*"We all worry about the population explosion,*
*but we don't worry about it at the right time."*

—Arthur Hoppe

## WHY BOTHER?

At one time, little girls had dreams of growing up to be mommies. Those dreams have changed considerably. Little girls know that they can be doctors, lawyers, presidents, and mommies. They are encouraged to become financially independent and career oriented, while being handed a Cabbage Patch Doll. Mixed messages of career, success, and procreation have created a need for young women to plan their lives carefully.

Preconceptional planning is the process of making changes in all areas of life before conception. This conscious planning will allow for a better pregnancy and parenting experience. Past generations felt that if they were able to conceive, then so be it. It was a blessing from God. While it may have been a blessing, it could also feel like a curse if other areas of the home life were unstable.

The timing of parenthood is probably what concerns today's women more than the actual changing role. Women are establishing their careers before undertaking marriage and children. It has become necessary for women to be driven employees and corporate ladder climbers. The trend is to be a superwoman in a critical and demanding business world. Women understand the urgency of planning for every move they make in their lives, and pregnancy is just another aspect that must be incorporated.

One of the basic areas to consider before pregnancy is the physical health of the mother-to-be. Changes in diet, weight, physical activities, and nutritional awareness are important considerations. A healthy body will give added assurance of a healthier pregnancy and baby.

Attitudes toward change play a vital role in preconceptional planning. Emotional and psychological considerations must be addressed.

The cute little baby in the stroller is rarely viewed as the "eighteen-year invader." While that may sound exaggerated, it is a reality of pregnancy and parenting. Babies are wonderful, exciting little people with many loving demands. They are helpless and remain dependent for years. Preparing for the demands of parenthood may require researching what life is really like with a new baby.

Babies do not fix relationships but rather reveal the existing strengths. A solid relationship or marriage is important before conception. Changes and strengthening in this area will create a more secure atmosphere for you as a couple and for the baby-to-be.

## BABY: A PERMANENT FIXTURE

Old movies portray young couples living on a shoestring and using a dresser drawer for their baby's crib. While Hollywood may have been able to portray this as a romantic situation, generating a few laughs, this sad lack of preparation is still common among new parents.

Men and women should examine their career choices with regard to the stability they possess. More women are returning to work after their maternity leave is over. What if the employer cannot guarantee the same position when she returns? Perhaps this is an area worth researching before conception. A career change may have to be considered. A man in the career world may be asked to uproot his family and move across the nation. Is this what he wants for his new family? This is also an area worth investigating.

Finances are a part of everyone's life. Couples are being faced with high interest rates on everything from houses and cars to charge cards. Financial awareness is an important area to consider before pregnancy occurs. Homeowning or renting, car buying or leasing, insurance policies, stocks, and bonds can all cause financial anxiety. Stable finances allow the couple planning a family to make a secure financial future for their child.

## WHAT IS RIGHT, WHAT IS WRONG?

With any decision to change, there is a question of the best approach. There will be areas of your life that need few adjustments and other areas that will need an overhaul. These changes are up to you; timing depends on your individual life schedule. As a tailored suit would not fit Jane if it were made for Jill, neither will life changes be the same for everyone.

2

Choosing what is right for you will make it workable for you. Changes are never easy, but if you persevere, you will succeed. Having realistic expectations for yourself is another vital ingredient in preconceptional planning. Placing a time frame on your changes will only create stress. That is something no one needs. Pregnancy planning is a time of self-examination, inside and out.

Making choices is a learned skill we develop as children. The choices we make as adults affect our world and those we know and love. Making preconceptional choices and changes are the first steps in parenting your child-to-be.

## JOE, JANE, JOHN, AND SALLY

Preparation for anything involves thought and planning. Very few people would consider having a formal dinner party without making formal plans. What would that be like?

Joe and Jane decide to have a party. On Friday at noon, they call fifty of their closest friends. They announce that they are having a sit-down dinner at 5:00 p.m. They then call Vinnie's Catering Service to order fifty-two complete lobster dinners. They call Guido's Furniture Rental to order chairs and a portable bar. Joe calls Bill and Bob's Beverage Bonanza to order beer, wine, and assorted liquors. Jane decides that it would be chic to have live entertainment, so she contacts the Velvet Violinists.

What do you suppose the reaction would have been in such a case of last-minute planning? Clearly, it would not have been possible for Joe and Jane to make these arrangements successfully. What is the difference between their last-minute preparation and not being ready for pregnancy? There is none. In both cases, planning ahead would allow for a more successful outcome.

Planning a pregnancy can also curtail the snowball effect that can occur. Sally and John have been married for two years. If Sally accidentally became pregnant, how would their life progress? Let's see.

Sally and her husband, John, live in an apartment complex that does not allow dogs, cats, or kids. First, they would have to find affordable housing before the baby arrives. John works with his brother and does not have major medical coverage. His benefits are limited and certainly do not include maternity or newborn care. Sally works in a factory where she is exposed to toxic chemicals. Her employer says he cannot make any accommodations for her just because she is pregnant. Sally

3

knows that these chemicals could harm her baby.

Sally and John have one truck that they must share to get to their jobs. Sally would have to go to her doctor's appointments more frequently as the pregnancy progresses. Of course, Sally and John live in a state that requires a baby car seat, but their pickup truck is not equipped for that. They may have to consider trading the truck for a car.

Sally is allowed six weeks of maternity leave after the baby is born. Because they rely on two incomes to pay the bills, Sally would have to find a baby-sitter. Their families live in other states, and they have very few friends. She would have to find a sitter who would agree to care for a newborn, which is difficult to do.

Sally is anxious about being pregnant, especially since she is only 20 years old. She and John both smoke and enjoy a beer with dinner every now and then. John says he is not going to change his life-style just because she is pregnant. Sally has been smoking since she was twelve and is not sure she wants to stop. After all, she is the one smoking, not the baby.

Sally and John have a multitude of changes that need to be made. It would have been of benefit for them to make these changes before pregnancy. Their situation is not uncommon, and because of an unplanned pregnancy, they are facing an avalanche of obstacles.

## FREE TO BE READY

Pregnancy is not a brick wall standing between a couple and changes. It limits changes by setting a time frame of nine months. It is never too late to begin improving the quality of life through change.

Women and couples need to view preconceptional planning as a liberation from complications. Addressing the various areas of pregnancy and parenting preconceptionally, parents-to-be are freeing their minds and energy for a happier pregnancy and birth experience.

Bertrand Russell once said, "The good life is one inspired by love and guided by knowledge." Deciding to make changes preconceptionally is the first step in loving the child-to-be. Increasing your knowledge so as to make choices is the second step. Both will allow you to give the good life to the life you are planning to create.

CHAPTER 2

# CHECKUPS BEGIN WITH YOU

*"Wherever the art of medicine is loved, there
also is love of humanity."*

—Hippocrates

## PROFESSIONAL OPINIONS

Preconception is the time to prepare for the stress and demands that
pregnancy places on the body. For most, the thought of purposely sub-
jecting themselves to a physical examination seems senseless. We tend to
wait until something is wrong before seeking our physician's help. For a
woman considering pregnancy, a physical is both practical and the most
basic of all considerations. If the health of the mother-to-be is compromised in any way, it may lead to complications.

A complete physical will reassure you that your body is in a healthy
state, ready for conception and pregnancy. There are certain medical
conditions that are not always compatible with pregnancy. Women with
chronic diseases should seek counseling from their doctor or specialists
concerning what pregnancy would hold for them.

Your family doctor will probably do a complete physical including
laboratory testing and a history of your health. These exams are tools to
evaluate your current health status and to aid your doctor in offering
advice that may improve your health.

The office or clinic nurse will probably be the first person to interview you. She will ask many questions, some that will require a few
moments of thought.

## WHAT A HISTORY

Questions, questions, and you have to supply the answers. Doctors call it
a "history." Here are some questions you may be asked:

- Name, address, telephone number, age, education, occupation,
  marital status, insurance coverage, and other personal details.
- Are both of your parents living? If not, what was their cause of

death? Are your sisters and brothers alive, and do they have any medical problems?

- Did you have any childhood diseases? Did you receive immunizations (baby shots) as a child?
- Did you ever have surgery? What for, when, where, and by whom?
- Are you allergic to anything?
- Do you have any medical problems that you are aware of?
- When did you have your first period? Have you ever been pregnant? If so, did you carry the pregnancy to full term?
- Are you presently taking any medications? If so, what for? Any prescription, nonprescription, or street drugs?
- Do you smoke? How many packs per day, and for how long?
- Do you drink? If so, how much a day, and for how long?

Medicine is like a puzzle. By asking questions and examining the facts, the doctor can figure out the best approach to your individual health goals.

## LET'S GET PHYSICAL

Pregnancy brings a variety of physical changes that will send the body on a roller coaster ride. If a woman has an unknown health problem, the stress of pregnancy will only make it worse. A physical examination, a gynecological assessment, and a dental checkup are where preconceptional planning begins.

A physical examination will include assessment of several areas. Evaluation of the heart and circulatory systems is easily performed. The doctor will listen to your heart, take a blood pressure reading, and ask questions specific to this body system. Because the fluid volume is increased by 40 percent in pregnancy, a healthy cardiac system is important.

The respiratory system, which includes the lungs, trachea (windpipe), sinuses, and nose, is examined. The doctor will listen to your lungs while asking you to take deep breaths in and out through your mouth. If there is a family history of asthma, emphysema, tuberculosis, or any other respiratory problems, tell your doctor. The lungs are compromised in pregnancy because of the growing uterus. Some women experience sinus problems such as congestion during pregnancy. It is important to have a healthy respiratory system for both you and your baby-to-be. Other body systems that will be examined include the nervous system, the gastrointestinal system (the stomach and bowels), bones and muscles, eyes, ears, nose, and throat, and the urinary system.

Laboratory testing may be performed on urine and blood samples. Some doctors collect these samples, while others send their patients to the hospital laboratory. The doctor receives the results from the lab. A chest X-ray may be ordered, and depending on the doctor's preference, he may order an electrocardiogram (EKG). An EKG is a test to evaluate the heart. Women who have a history of heart problems or irregular heartbeats may be asked to undergo one.

To obtain that clean bill of health and feel good about conceiving, a visit with the family doctor is a worthwhile trip.

## Routine Laboratory Tests

### Blood Tests

| | |
|---|---|
| *Blood Type* | To determine blood type in case a blood transfusion is needed. |
| *Rh Factor* | The Rh is the + or − of the blood type. Rh+ includes 85 percent of the population, without complication. Rh-, however, is of concern to a woman considering pregnancy. If her baby is Rh+, then her body may become sensitive and produce Rh antibodies that would affect subsequent pregnancies, causing damage to future fetuses. |
| *Hemoglobin and Hematocrit* | Hemoglobin in the blood carries oxygen throughout the body. Hematocrit is the percentage of erythrocytes, or mature red blood cells, in a given volume of blood. While levels may be low in pregnancy, abnormally low levels require treatment. |
| *Rubella Titer* | Rubella, or German measles, is a virus that can be dangerous to pregnant women because of its damage to the baby. A titer shows if a woman has been immunized against Rubella. If she has not, it is suggested that she do so before conception, allowing at least three months between immunization and conception. |

7

| | |
|---|---|
| *RPR* | Rapid Plasma Reagin test indicates the presence of syphilis. Early detection allows for treatment before pregnancy. |
| *Glucose* | This test is used to indicate the ability of the body to adjust adequately to carbohydrate metabolism. Pregnancy adds a stress to the body and may even cause a disorder called gestational diabetes. If there is an existing glucose intolerance, it may be picked up before conception. |

| | |
|---|---|
| **Urine Tests** *Urinalysis* | This test is performed to assess the kidney's ability to filter and dispose of waste products. |
| *Albumin* | Checking for protein in the urine is a common test during pregnancy. A strip of special paper is dipped into the urine and changes color according to what it monitors. The amount of protein in the urine shows the body's ability to maintain fluid levels throughout the body. Conditions like toxemia are monitored during pregnancy by this test. |

| | |
|---|---|
| **Vaginal Tests** *Pap Smear* | This test is performed to diagnose any cervical abnormality that may indicate the possibility of cancer. The care giver swabs the cervix and places the smear on a slide to be viewed by the laboratory. |

## Sexually Transmitted Diseases

Each year ten million Americans acquire some form of sexually transmitted disease. They are passed primarily through sexual contact. They are passed between men and women and between men. It is not enough to be a "good girl," especially if you are someone who enjoys sex. Safe sex is a great concept, but spontaneity and desire remain overwhelming factors. The fact remains that these diseases are dangerous. The most common are gonorrhea, genital herpes, genital warts, syphilis, and chlamydia.

The greatest danger with these diseases is neglecting to seek treatment. Receiving treatment may prevent a future filled with complications that are health related. Several of these diseases can lead to sterility in both women and their partners. The woman considering pregnancy must be certain that she and her partner are disease-free.

## Chlamydia
Women may experience a thin vaginal discharge or cystitis. Symptoms are few. Men will have a discharge from the penis and painful urination. A culture is taken of the discharge from the cervix. For men, a culture is also obtained. Tetracycline is the drug of choice. In addition, the use of condoms is recommended until both are free of infection.

## Gonorrhea
Women show signs of infection two to eight days after exposure. Symptoms are burning on urination and a vaginal discharge. Men may have a thick, milky discharge from the penis and severe burning when urinating.

The cervix is swabbed for a culture of the discharge. A discharge from the man is tested. High doses of injectable penicillin are generally prescribed. Oral ampicillin or amoxicillin may be used in high doses as well.

## Genital Herpes
Symptoms are painful sores around the sex organs. Sores are blisters or clusters of blisters.

Diagnosis is made with a direct examination by a doctor and laboratory tests of tissue samples and blood. There is no treatment since genital herpes is caused by a virus. Symptom relief is obtained by use of aloe vera gel to soothe and dry sores.

## Genital Warts
Resembling regular warts, genital warts may be seen three weeks to three months after exposure. Women may notice them on the vaginal lips, on the inside of the vagina, or on the cervix or anus. Men will see them at the tip of the penis or around the foreskin.

Direct examination is performed by a doctor. They may be diagnosed by an abnormal PAP smear, a biopsy of tissue, or by open sores.

Podophyllin solution or a variety of other acidic solutions are applied. Cryotherapy, or freezing off, is an alternative. Electrodesiccation, or burning off the warts, is also a treatment. All of these procedures are done by a doctor.

## Syphilis

Symptoms appear 10 to 90 days after contact. Sores appear on the genitalia or the mouth and may disappear and recur repeatedly. There may be a rash, low fever, or a sore throat.

A culture of discharge from sores is taken for diagnosis. On the disappearance of the sores, a blood test determines infection. Injection of penicillin is the treatment of choice.

## Acquired Immune Deficiency Syndrome

AIDS is not just a disease of the gay population. The sad truth is that men, women, and children are all potential victims. The preconceptional woman is faced with the decision to request a blood test to determine if she has been exposed to the virus.

The human immunodeficiency virus (HIV) is transmitted by infected blood or semen. It can enter the body through intercourse, either vaginal or rectal. The virus also can enter through oral sex. Another way is through sharing a needle for intravenous (IV) drug use. One may also be infected through contaminated blood transfusions. HIV is transmitted between men and women, men and men, and mother and unborn child. HIV crosses the placenta usually in the first three months of pregnancy. Approximately 75 percent of the HIV positive children acquired the virus while in their mothers' wombs.

A positive HIV test does not necessarily mean an active infection of AIDS. The virus causes the body to lose its ability to fight off other diseases and may live in the body for years before symptoms are manifested.

Testing is available and should be requested for anyone who is not sure if she has been exposed to the virus. Knowing your partner is important. Ask him his sexual history and recall your own to attempt to eliminate any questions. If you are in doubt, seek help from your family doctor or a clinic.

Prevention is still the best reassurance you have. If you are planning to become sexually active with someone you do not know, hand him a condom.

If you are an IV drug user, get help. Quitting may be the most important decision you will ever make. Besides the obvious destruction to your body, AIDS is an ever-present threat. Sharing needles can only lead to sharing diseases. AIDS is a disease for which there is no cure.

## The Gynecological Examination

Any woman who is planning to conceive should seek professional guidance. This can be accomplished by locating a family doctor who handles gynecology and obstetrics, a certified nurse midwife, or an obstetrician/gynecologist. (See chap. 15.)

Whomever you choose, here are a few considerations:

- Is this the person you want to be active in the delivery of your baby, once you have conceived?
- On an emergency basis, will this doctor or midwife see you or will one of her partners, if she is in a group practice?
- Does this care giver share your philosophies about preparing for pregnancy, prenatal care, labor procedures, and interventions?
- Is the hospital at which your care giver practices reputable, with current standards in obstetrical care for its patients?
- Consider interviewing care givers before committing yourself to one. Ask other women whom they see and compare notes. It is a wise decision to shop around.

A typical gynecological examination will include the following:

### An Interview

An interview will include your personal and family medical history. Sometimes specific gynecological questions concerning your mother and sisters may be asked. You will also have to know when you began menstruation, how long your period lasts, and if you have any problems with your cycle.

### Physical Examination

This includes examination of the breasts and the external genitals as well as an internal pelvic examination and a rectal examination.

### *Breast Examination*

The breasts are composed of fat, connective tissue, and mammary glands that produce milk. Breasts begin developing at adolescence. From that point on, hormones will influence the size of breasts at different stages in a woman's life. It is important for you to examine your breasts each month for any cystic (hard) areas, or lumps. Your care giver will check your breasts and, if you wish, will show you how.

Monthly breast examinations are simple to perform and may save your life. Early detection of lumps by regular examinations will allow you to receive treatment before a malignancy can spread.

### External Genitalia
This includes the area from the pubic bone to the perineum (the area between the vagina and rectum). This includes the labia, clitoris, urethra (urinary opening), and vaginal opening. By examining these areas, your physician can spot any abnormalities and treat them, if necessary.

### Cervical Examination
After the external organs have been checked, the care giver will examine the vagina and the cervix. The cervix is checked for abnormalities and a Pap test is performed.

Pap is short for Papanicolaou, the doctor who discovered that cancerous tumors of the uterus and cervix shed their cells. By testing the cervical area, problems can be detected.

Women are encouraged to be tested yearly. Women who take birth control pills should be tested twice a year. If there is any sign of changing cells, your care giver will inform you and can treat the condition before conception occurs.

### Bimanual Exam
The care giver places her gloved and lubricated fingers into the vaginal canal. She then pushes up with that hand, while pushing down on your abdomen with the other hand. She is pushing your uterus down and keeping your cervix in place to feel its shape and position. She will also feel both ovaries and fallopian tubes. This will give her an idea of what the reproductive organs are like and if they feel normal.

### Rectal Exam
This examination will allow the care giver to feel the back of the uterus and cervix. It is done with a gloved hand. The care giver inserts her index finger into the vagina and her middle finger into the rectum. While pushing down from the abdomen with the other hand, she can feel the cervix and uterus from another angle. This part of the exam is not particularly comfortable, but it is important.

## Dental Examination
Preventive health care is carried into the dental office as well. Pregnancy affects the condition of teeth. There is an increased incidence of dental caries (cavities) and gum infections. Some women experience

swelling of the gums accompanied by bleeding. This occurs because of an increase in hormone production.

A thorough checkup by your dentist before conception will allow for necessary treatment. Fillings, extractions, root canal, and, of course, X-rays can be safely performed. Major dental work requiring general anesthesia can be safely performed before conception. Brushing after every meal, flossing, and rinsing with a mouthwash should help keep bacteria to a minimum. Maintenance of a good diet high in calcium and Vitamin C will also contribute to healthy teeth.

## Preexisting Medical Conditions

Technological advances have turned disappointing futures into hopeful outlooks for women with chronic diseases. For example, it was once considered impossible for a diabetic woman to conceive. Now, not only is she able to conceive but with close observation by her care giver, she is able to carry her baby for a full-term pregnancy.

Women who have chronic disorders who are considering pregnancy have some special things to consider. The following are just a few common medical conditions and how pregnancy affects them.

### Bronchial Asthma

Asthma is a respiratory illness that can be aggravated by things like temperature changes, allergens, or emotional tension. Asthma attacks cause a constriction of the windpipe, not allowing adequate oxygen to reach the lungs. Anyone with a history of asthma knows how to avoid some of the things that cause an attack. On occasion, however, it is unavoidable. Medication is available and either taken in pill form or by inhaler. This dilates the bronchial tubes that have closed off the airway.

A woman considering pregnancy should be sure to inform her allergist or doctor of her plans. Medications can cross the placenta and affect the baby. The effect of pregnancy on women with asthma is difficult to foretell. Be sure to discuss with your doctor how he plans to handle the asthma and pregnancy for a positive outcome.

### Epilepsy

This neurological disorder complicates one out of 1,000 pregnancies. It is a disorder that is most commonly known for the seizures that follow a temporary disturbance in the brain's impulses. The seizures vary in severity from one person to another.

Epileptics are usually on medication to help with seizure control. Anticonvulsant drugs like Dilantin are generally used. A woman considering pregnancy should understand that Dilantin is harmful to the fetus. Drugs like Valium and Librium are safe. Complications of pregnancy such as edema, low calcium, and low blood sugar can increase the likelihood of convulsions.

Epilepsy is not an indication to avoid pregnancy, nor does it mean ending an existing pregnancy. It is also felt there is no need to avoid labor and a vaginal delivery. The epileptic woman should carefully consider pregnancy with the understanding that outcomes are unpredictable. The good news is that women are taking care of themselves and their fetuses under the watchful eye of their care giver and are having positive outcomes.

### Multiple Sclerosis

MS is a disease that is identified by hardened patches scattered throughout the brain and spinal cord. These patches interfere with the nerves in those areas. It is extremely disabling and includes periods of improvement and worsening. Symptoms include weakening and tremors of the limbs as well as a slurring of the speech. There may be an unsteady gait and even the potential of loss of bladder and bowel control.

MS frequently presents itself initially after a pregnancy and is more common during the childbearing years. It may complicate pregnancy in an MS patient.

Women with this disorder may actually be at an advantage, however. It is possible to have an almost pain-free delivery. Careful consideration of pregnancy before it occurs should be undertaken with the guidance of your doctor.

### Systemic Lupus Erythematosus

This is a disease that falls under the group known as collagen disorders. What occurs in Lupus is a deterioration of the connective tissues in various parts of the body. It may attack the soft internal organs, the bones, and the muscles. It may even be fatal. It is often treated with corticosteroids to control the symptoms.

It most commonly affects women of childbearing age. If a woman with lupus decides to become pregnant, she is advised to wait two years after the diagnosis and until the disease is under control with medication. The obstetrician will observe the cardiovascular and renal systems carefully. Steroid therapy is continued throughout the pregnancy, including steroids administered intravenously during labor and delivery.

## Rheumatoid Arthritis

This is a disease that affects one out of 100 Americans. Three-fourths of those affected are women, with the usual age for onset between 20 and 50 years old. It is an autoimmune disorder, meaning that the immune system works against the body. There is pain, stiffness, tenderness, and swelling of the joints.

Seventy-five percent of the women who have rheumatoid arthritis and become pregnant notice a decrease in the severity of their symptoms. This is due to the increase in hormone levels. Although this is good news, the symptoms will return about one month after delivery. Medications are discontinued during the last three months of pregnancy and after delivery if the mother is breast feeding. Women with total joint replacements in the hips and knees have experienced successful vaginal deliveries with healthy babies.

The woman with rheumatoid arthritis should make careful plans before conception. She should discuss them with her rheumatologist or orthopedist and her obstetrical care giver.

## Cardiovascular Disorders

Heart disease affects one-half to 2 percent of pregnant women. Conditions that may cause heart disease include rheumatic fever, syphilis, arteriosclerosis, and, of course, congenital malformations. Whatever the cause, these women who desire to become pregnant should consult a cardiologist.

Pregnancy places an additional work load on the heart. It increases the heart rate by 15 to 20 beats in the last three months of pregnancy and stimulates a 40 percent increase in blood volume. A normal heart is able to compensate for the additional stress. The diseased heart may find it difficult to handle the strain of pregnancy, labor, and delivery. The possibility of surgical correction of any congenital malformation should be discussed with the cardiologist. Before you conceive is the time to have this done.

Some areas of special consideration are the following:
• Prenatal checkups may be more frequent and more detailed.
• A strict diet high in iron and protein must be followed.
• If ordered by the doctor, bed rest must be undertaken.

15

- Stresses of home, job, and environment must be eliminated.
- Infections must be avoided to prevent endocarditis. The administration of penicillin may be prescribed to prevent this.
- If a woman is taking any medications for her heart, like a blood thinner, she will need to discuss its effect on the baby with her doctor.
- The woman must understand that depending on the severity of her heart disease, her labor and delivery may involve considerable intervention. Delivery may include the use of forceps to prevent the extreme stress of pushing in the final stage of labor.

The woman with heart disease has quite a decision to make. With the help of her doctor, she will be able to do what is realistic for her medical condition.

## Diabetes

Before the discovery of insulin, many diabetic girls died before reaching puberty. Those who did survive were either sterile or did not menstruate. If pregnancy did occur, there was a 25 percent maternal death rate and a 50 percent fetal and newborn death rate.

Improvements in technology, diagnosis, and management of the diabetic woman have increased the incidence of conception and delivery of children. Although there is improvement in the outcome of a well-managed diabetic pregnancy, a certain risk to the newborn remains.

Pregnancy requires the body to make alterations in metabolism. The diabetic woman is dealing with an existing alteration in her body's ability to process carbohydrates. The pancreas is not functioning properly, so there is an insulin deficiency. Pregnancy requires that the body make adjustments as the baby grows.

During the first trimester, months 1-3 of pregnancy, the baby uses its mother's glucose. This lowers her need to produce as much insulin. Throughout the second trimester, months 4-9, the baby uses more of the mother's glucose to match its own insulin production. After delivery, the circulating hormones, steroids, and insulin levels drop off. The mother's pancreas rapidly adjusts and returns to its prepregnant state. These normal changes occur smoothly without notice in a woman with a healthy pancreas.

For the diabetic mother, there are special considerations to be made for pregnancy. Dietary management or insulin control should be based on the woman's glucose levels. Diet should be tailored with the help of a registered dietician. Weight gain should be discussed with the dietician and the care giver.

Regular exercise should continue, with the diabetic mother-to-be adjusting her diet and insulin accordingly. Insulin-dependent women will need to discuss with their care giver how they plan to adjust their insulin doses. With the development of Autolet, the device used for finger sticks at home, the woman can determine her blood glucose level and make the needed insulin adjustments.

Office visits may be as frequent as every two weeks for the first 32 weeks of pregnancy, then weekly until delivery. The usual prenatal assessment is done, with the addition of extra monitoring of urine and blood levels.

Pregnancy is a demanding state for a healthy body. The diabetic woman should decide if pregnancy is realistic for her. It is a challenge; and yet because of technology and determined young women, it can be an achievable dream.

## Physically Challenged Women

Several million women in this country are holding jobs, going to school, becoming mothers, and changing the world. These women are paralyzed, blind, deaf, or compromised in other physical areas. They are, however, on the move and unable to be content simply existing. These women also consider pregnancy and parenting as options in their lives.

Physically challenged women should follow the same planning preconceptionally, including a physical examination, a gynecological examination, and an evaluation of their particular disability and how pregnancy and parenting will affect it.

Women who are paralyzed are able to become pregnant depending on their health. Labor and delivery will need to be addressed individually. The pain of labor may not be felt, but forceps may be used during the pushing stage of delivery. Caring for her newborn will be challenging for the paraplegic woman but not impossible.

Deaf women considering pregnancy should be aware of the adjustments needed with the addition of a child. Most important will be including a system in the home to indicate if the baby is crying. Technological advances have made hearing loss almost void of impairment. Lights and other visual aids are available to assist the hearing-impaired woman. Children of deaf parents have no difficulty communicating.

They are exposed to TV, radio, friends, and family members who are not deaf, and they may learn sign language as well.

Women who are visually impaired have minor adjustments to make in the consideration of pregnancy and parenting. Because of the increase in development of her other senses, the blind mother is able to perform all areas of child care that a sighted mother does. It is helpful if the mother has a strong support system. The woman's doctor should be supportive and sensitive to her special needs. She should follow the same preconceptional planning, making adjustments needed for the addition of the baby.

Physical challenges are just another area of a woman's life. It is vital to establish realistic expectations of what pregnancy and parenting mean to the physically challenged woman. While family and friends may not always be supportive of such an undertaking, the decision is yours.

Establishing a baseline assessment of your health will allow for the next step, that of making changes. A physical examination will assure you all systems are in good health. The gynecological examination will determine the likelihood of a successful conception. The laboratory testing will give your care giver an idea of what areas of your body need special treatment or improvement. With your doctor's assistance, you can now begin to explore what changes will create a healthier body for you.

## SUGGESTED READING

*Every Woman's Health: The Couple's Guide to Body and Mind*
D. S. Thompson
Doubleday, revised and expanded, 1985

*The Herpes Handbook*
Terri Gunn and Mary Stenzel-Poore
VD Action Council
OHSU-L220A
Portland, OR 97201

*Herpes in Pregnancy*
Pennypress, Inc.
1100 23rd Avenue East
Seattle, WA 98112
Cost: 1-5 copies at 50 cents each

*The A-Z of Women's Health: A Concise Encyclopedia*
Christine Ammer
Everest House, 1983

*Woman Care: A Gynecological Guide to Your Body*
Lynda Madaras, and Jane Patterson, M.D.
Avon Books, 1981

*Outwitting Arthritis*
Isabel Hanson
Creative Arts Book Co., 1980
833 Bancroft Way
Berkeley, CA 94710

*The Arthritis Exercise Book*
Semyon Krewer
Simon and Schuster, 1981

*The Diabetics' Total Health Book*
June Biermand and Barbara Toohey
J. P. Tarcher, 1980

*Lupus and Pregnancy*
Pennsylvania Lupus Foundation
P.O. Box 264
Wayne, PA 19087

*Lupus Facts*
Lupus Erythematosus Foundation
Boston, MA 02108

## RESOURCE GROUPS

The National Multiple Sclerosis Society
257 Park Avenue South
New York, NY 10010
212-986-3240

The Epilepsy Foundation of America
733 15th Street
Washington, D.C. 20005
301-459-3700

Juvenile Diabetes Foundation International
Hotline: 1-800-223-1137
New York: 1-212-889-8174
Answers questions.

Public Health Service
AIDS Information Hotline
1-800-342-AIDS
Alaska and Hawaii only: Call collect 202-245-6867
Information to the public.

National Diabetes Information Clearinghouse
Box NDIC
Bethesda, MD 20205
301-468-2162

Arthritis Information Clearinghouse
Box 9782
Arlington, VA 22209
703-558-8250

American Heart Association
7320 Greenville Avenue
Dallas, TX 75231
214-373-6300

VD Hotline
Operation Venus
1-800-982-5883
Provides free and confidential information on STD.

CHAPTER 3

# INTERNAL CONDITIONING
## Healthy Dieting Just for You

*"Americans: People who laugh at. . .African witch doctors
and spend 100 million dollars on fake reducing systems."*
— Leonard Louis Levinson

## NUTRITION IN A NUTSHELL

Women and men all over the world have become health conscious. It is
not enough for those concerned to get their bodies in shape on the outside and neglect the inside. Women thinking about pregnancy have an
even more important consideration. Only 20 to 30 percent of women in
the United States begin pregnancy in a good nutritional state.

What can be said about nutrition that has not appeared in every
woman's magazine, in TV commercials, or on bookshelves? Not much.
For the preconceptional woman, good eating is more than just a casual
concept. It is the basis for building a life.

Good nutrition is important for both mother and baby. Once a
woman becomes aware of food content, like nutrients, vitamins, and
minerals, she can be assured her unborn child will have a healthy start.
The American College of Obstetricians and Gynecologists issued the
following statement concerning nutrition and pregnancy: "A woman's
nutritional status before, during, and after pregnancy contributes to a
significant degree to the well-being of both herself and her infant.
Therefore, what a woman consumes before she conceives and while she
carries the fetus is of vital importance to the health of succeeding generations."

With that in mind, the woman considering pregnancy can see why
the establishment of healthy eating patterns is important. The changes
that occur during pregnancy include hormonal, physical, and biochemi-
cal. These changes determine the need for nutrients and how the body
uses them.

In 1977, the U. S. Senate Select Committee on Nutrition and Human
Needs published dietary goals for Americans. They suggested some of
the following changes:

- Eat more fresh fruits, vegetables, and whole grains.
- Substitute skim milk or low-fat milk for full-fat milk, except for infants and children.
- Eat less animal fat.
- Eat less refined sugar and fewer foods high in refined sugar.
- Eat fewer high-cholesterol foods.
- Eat fewer high-fat foods.
- Eat less salt and fewer salty foods.

Although we believe we are a well-informed nation, our eating habits leave a lot to be desired. To truly nourish our bodies, we must understand what foods are helpful.

## GOOD FOOD VERSUS BAD FOOD

What is good food and what is bad food? Pizza and popcorn were once thought of as junk foods. We have come to understand that when made with a whole-wheat crust, tomato sauce, cheese, and perhaps sausage or hamburger, a pizza is a complete meal. And popcorn is now the snack most preferred by parents for their kids. Adults love it as well, since plain popcorn is low in calories.

Understanding what is needed to fuel and nourish these machines we call bodies is what good eating is all about. Some basic substances are vital for growth and survival.

### Protein

When you think of proteins, picture a child playing with blocks. He takes a few blocks and creates a foundation. Then, he places a few more blocks on the base and begins the walls. Protein acts as the support, the foundation, and the frame of our cells of life.

The structure of muscles, connective tissues, and various glands depend on the existence of protein. Babies are built, children grow, wounds heal, and muscle mass is increased by this basic substance.

Protein can be found in both animal and vegetable forms. Our society is well off in its protein intake. Some foods that provide protein are:

- Legumes, like lentils, peas, pinto beans, soybeans, chickpeas, and kidney beans.
- Meat, milk, yogurt, eggs, fish, and poultry.
- Nuts, sesame seeds, sunflower seeds, peanuts, and peanut butter.
- Grains, whole wheat, oats, rye, wheat germ, wheat bran, brown rice, and whole grain pasta.

A pregnant woman needs almost 70 percent more protein. The preconceptional woman can begin to build her protein intake from the variety of choices available.

## Vitamins

A normal healthy woman, eating a well-balanced, healthy diet, probably does not need a supplemental vitamin. The key words are "well-balanced" and "healthy." Today's women are working either at home or away from home. Either way, chances are slim that her meals occur at regular intervals and are well balanced. A woman of childbearing age and older should be taking a multivitamin with iron to pick up where her diet fails.

Pregnancy requires a good supply of certain vitamins and minerals to assure a healthy pregnancy and baby. Some of them are as follows.

### Fat-Soluble Vitamins

These vitamins are stored in the body's fat supply.

### Vitamin A

This vitamin plays a part in building resistance to infection. It also aids in the development of tooth enamel and bone development. It is found in green, leafy vegetables as well as orange vegetables and fruits. It is found in organ meats, butter, and whole or fortified milk. Spinach, kale, beets, watercress, dandelion greens, and cantaloupes are all rich suppliers of Vitamin A.

### Vitamin D

This particular vitamin is increased by simply sitting in the sun. The sun's ultraviolet rays interact with the oils of the skin, producing Vitamin D, which is then absorbed into the body through the pores. Beware, however, once you have that golden tan, further absorption of Vitamin D stops. It is an important vitamin for healthy bones and teeth. It is found in fortified milk, tuna, salmon, and liver. Other foods that include D are margarine and dairy products.

### Water Soluble Vitamins

These vitamins are excreted in the urine.

23

## B Vitamins

There are eleven different vitamins under the heading of the "Bs." They work together, aiding each other in their individual performances. The group includes riboflavin, thiamine, folic acid, B6, and pantothenic acid.

This group of vitamins produces a number of effects on the body. Their basic benefits include prevention of skin problems, preventing nervousness, and providing energy. They help extract energy from the carbohydrates, proteins, and fats we consume. The Bs help build body tissues like mucous membranes. In pregnancy, they play an important role in cell division, fetal growth, and the prevention of anemia.

Some foods high in the B vitamins include whole grains, wheat germ, milk, nuts, organ meats, and mushrooms as well as green and leafy vegetables.

## Vitamin C

Essential for wound healing, this vitamin can be found in many different enjoyable foods. It also helps decrease or eliminate bruising or bleeding gums. Citrus fruits, tomatoes, peppers, broccoli, cantaloupes, cabbage, and strawberries are some of the foods rich in C.

This vitamin is not stored in our bodies, so it must be supplied daily. In pregnancy, it helps with the development of teeth and bones, a healthy placenta, and strong cell and blood vessel walls. Establishing a daily supply of Vitamin C may be as simple as drinking a glass of orange juice or taking a supplement that includes C. Keep in mind while cooking any foods rich in C, that heat will destroy the vitamin, decreasing the food's C content.

## Major Minerals

### Calcium

Calcium is a form of insurance for the woman preparing for pregnancy. By building a supply before conception, you and your baby will have your calcium needs met.

Osteoporosis and calcium intake are the latest in women's health issues. While there is merit in supplementing to avoid osteoporosis, there is an urgency in doing so preconceptionally. If a pregnant woman does not take adequate amounts of calcium, the fetus will take it from her supply. This can lead to leg cramps. Other benefits of calcium include aiding in the absorption of Vitamin B12 and clotting of blood. It builds the baby's bones and teeth while in the uterus.

Calcium can be found in a variety of foods and drinks. The number of nontraditional foods that contain calcium may surprise you. Here are some sources for calcium.

- Milk and its products.
- Yogurt, cheddar and Swiss cheese, and buttermilk for easier digestion.
- Acidophilus milk, which contains predigested lactose for those with a milk intolerance.
- Soybeans, and other legumes, almonds, and sesame seeds.
- Figs, apricots, and dates.
- Broccoli, kale, rhubarb, dark greens, and okra.
- Oysters, canned salmon, sardines with bones, and shrimp.

A 50 percent increase in calcium intake is required during pregnancy. A variety of foods, as well as supplements in pill form, are available.

## Iron

Dieting, menstruation, and poor eating habits are leading causes of an inadequate supply of iron. Anemia can develop, leading to weakness and chronic fatigue.

Iron is a vital mineral to assure a healthy blood supply for both mother and baby-to-be. It is important for developing hemoglobin, which carries oxygen in the blood. Women of childbearing age and older should consider taking an iron supplement. During pregnancy, a well-established iron supply is important. The mother accumulates iron stores, which she, in turn, passes to her baby. The iron that is passed from mother to child then supplies the baby with enough of the mineral to last for the first few months of life.

Iron-rich foods include the following:

- Meats: organ meats like liver, heart, and kidney as well as beef.
- Prunes, dried apricots, prune juice, and raisins.
- Wheat germ, dried beans, and tofu.
- Oysters.
- Dark green vegetables like spinach, kale, endive, and broccoli.
- Whole or enriched grain foods.
- Even cooking in cast-iron pots helps increase the iron content of foods.

## WEIGHT: OVER OR UNDER?

Weight is controlled by food intake, exercise, and inherited body size. Women are bombarded by social standards encouraging them to look like models. What we do not realize is that we are not meant to look like shapeless, undernourished pictures. What is right for your body may not be right for someone else's. With that in mind, women should examine what is realistic and important in weight control for a healthier body.

There are standards for what is considered ideal body weight (IBW). Height, bone size, and age are assessed to determine an individual's IBW. It is important to realize that it is possible to be underweight. Starving the body destroys life and can actually prevent conception. Women who have chosen purposely to starve themselves suffer from anorexia nervosa. Another syndrome, known as bulimia, is also a hazardous disorder. Women will eat excessively and then purge themselves by vomiting or with laxatives. Either disorder is dangerous and can lead to death. Women with these disorders have more than just a problem with their food intake. Quite often, it is an expression of extreme self-denial, of repression of conflict or anger, or of control. By controlling her weight and image, she feels in control of what may be a life otherwise out of control.

For the sake of an image, we may be starving our bodies, preventing ourselves from conceiving when we desire. The human body has a way of preserving itself. When vital organs are in need of the body's energies, the body will shut down such systems as the reproductive system, which is not vital to maintain life. Women quite often experience a missed period when they are under stress or have a chronic illness. The same goes for suboptimal nutrition. The body has enough sense to know that it could not adequately handle pregnancy and sustain life for itself. Pregnancy in these cases often does not occur.

Whichever challenge you choose, to lose or gain weight, be sure to set realistic goals for yourself. If you want to gain weight, what is the best strategy for gaining without overloading with the wrong types of foods? If you want to lose weight, what should be your goal? The most important thing to remember is to adjust your weight before conception to assure a successful conception and a healthy body for pregnancy.

### Diet Now, Not Later

Weight loss is part exercise and part diet modification. Dieting has become an American obsession. There are various diets ranging from eating grapefruit to eating all the brownies you can in a weekend. Some diets will aid in losing weight. But will they sustain weight loss after the diet is over?

To establish a diet that is safe and reliable, the family doctor should be consulted. Some of the factors to take into consideration are these:

Is your weight in proportion according to the standards set by the American Dietetic Association?

Will the diet your doctor suggests fit into your life-style? If not, can he help you decide how to work around it and still reach your dietary goals?

Does your doctor suggest a vitamin and mineral supplement to replace what may be lost during dieting? If not, what is the reason for not supplementing?

Does the doctor suggest exercise to accompany your diet? Can he suggest what types are best for burning calories?

If your doctor prescribes diet pills, does that mean a "crutch" until you lose weight? Will pills assure a sustained weight loss, or will weight be regained after the pills are stopped? When would it be safe to attempt conception after stopping the diet pills?

Dieting for your benefit as well as your baby's is a wise decision. It will be profitable for a lifetime. Reaching your dietary goals one step at a time is a rewarding accomplishment.

## Dieting Strategies

Robert Quillen had this to say about diet strategies: "Another good reducing exercise consists in placing both hands against the table edge and pushing back." Diets, exercise, medications, and willpower are all different techniques for decreasing weight.

Diets vary from low carbohydrate to low fat to low protein to grape-fruit. There are diets that are combined with support groups and diets that involve no food at all.

A diet plan that is nutritionally sound and involves support is Weight Watchers. Group support settings tend to be the most successful for treating weight loss as people in group settings are inclined to stay in the program longer and are more likely to lose weight. Encouragement from others with a mutual goal is a positive approach both physically and psychologically.

Behavior modification is just that. Modifying your eating habits is a learned behavior. It can be done in several ways:

- Eat while seated at a proper eating place and using knives, spoons, and forks.
- Concentrate on eating.
- Plan menus.
- Eat slowly, chew slowly, and pause between bites.
- Do your grocery shopping after you have eaten, and always use a list.

## Diet Drugs

Medications used to treat overweight individuals are not always effective and may be dangerous. There are several types of drugs. Some suppress the appetite, some increases the body's metabolic rate, and some are diuretics.

Appetite suppressants are also known as anorectic drugs. They contain the same properties found in the hormones adrenaline and noradrenaline. The most common drug is amphetamine, which has unfavorable side effects. Some of these are a decrease in fatigue, an increase in alertness, and a feeling of euphoria. While these do not sound like negative side effects, in reality, the user is unable to know just how tired she really is. It is a false sense of burning calories. Insomnia is a side effect that could severely interfere with work performance and safety. There is weight loss with these medications, but the ability to sustain weight control is inadequate once the medication is stopped.

The weight loss with calorigenic drugs seems impressive. The problem with these medications is that they cause an increase in oxygen consumption. Protein as opposed to fat is actually burned. Protein is needed by the body to make muscle. There can be cardiac problems from taking these drugs.

Diuretics are used to rid the body of excessive fluids. Women who retain fluid in their body tissues may see a temporary dramatic weight loss. The fat stores are not affected by diuretics. These drugs can also lead to side effects harmful to the cardiac system. One of these is the loss of potassium through excessive urination. Potassium keeps the heart muscle beating at a regular smooth rate. If the body loses too much potassium, it can cause an irregular heartbeat.

Diet drugs are only temporary crutches that cannot guarantee sustained weight loss. They threaten the body with complications.

Everything from protein diets, fasting, skipping meals, drugs, surgery, and jaw wiring can help you lose weight, or so they claim. Whatever strategy you choose, make sure it is realistic for your life-style. If your goal includes keeping the weight off, be sure to include a sport and exercise program.

## Diet Demons

Nothing can ruin efforts to become internally conditioned more than the "demons of dieting": caffeine, alcohol, drugs, and tobacco.

### Caffeine

Caffeine is one of those drugs that can be found hiding in foods and drinks. You can bet Mr. Hershey never thought twice about marketing those heavenly chocolate bars. Although that cup of coffee is "good to the last drop," too much can be bad news.

Caffeine is found in colas, chocolate, coffees, teas, and over-the-counter pain relievers. Animal studies show the possibility of birth defects and low birth weights associated with high caffeine consumption by pregnant women.

Helpful substitutes like unsweetened fruit juices and herbal teas are natural alternatives for that early morning java. Raisins, nuts, and seeds are excellent snacks to replace that chocolate bar at break time. This may require some planning ahead and taking your own snacks and beverages to work.

Liberating your body from caffeine is not an easy task. It is an addiction. Slow withdrawal is a practical technique. You may experience headaches and irritability. Remain true to your goal, and be gentle with yourself. Preparing your body for conception means this demon must go.

### Alcohol

Seventy percent of American women drink some form of alcohol. Whether it is a beer with a meal or a bottle of vodka every other day, most women are alcohol consumers.

Alcohol produces no positive effects on the health of a drinker. It damages the liver and brain, two organs that are irreplaceable. The tragic effect of alcohol occurs when a pregnant woman drinks.

There is no known safe level of alcohol a pregnant woman can consume. The likelihood of miscarriage during the second trimester (months 4, 5, and 6) increases for women who drink one to two alcoholic beverages or more per day. If spontaneous abortion does not occur, an abnormal baby may be born. The most common abnormalities include head and facial defects, abnormal arms and legs, and problems with the genitourinary system as well as the heart. Such babies may have a low birth weight and any number of behavioral defects like jitteriness, a decrease in alertness, poor sucking ability, and sleep and feeding difficulties.

The effects of drinking during pregnancy can follow a child throughout his life. Because of damage to the central nervous system, some children of women who drink during pregnancy have mild to moderate behavioral and learning deficiencies.

If you are considering pregnancy and find you are addicted to alcohol, seek help. Alcohol benefits no one. It destroys the good you have decided to do for your body. For every drink you take, you defeat the purpose of internal conditioning.

Like other habits or dependencies, alcohol controls our lives and bodies. It is not an easy habit to break, and it may require help from other people. A self-help program should include other drinkers, for example, Alcoholics Anonymous (AA).

AA has been in existence for over 60 years and has been the beginning of true living for thousands of men and women alcoholics. This organization is located in every state and city. It is as simple as looking in the telephone book and making a call. Choosing to stop drinking is one of the healthiest life-style changes that can be made.

Pregnancy and alcohol are contradictory terms. One creates life, the other destroys it. Quitting drinking is the first step to increase the chances of a healthy pregnancy and baby.

### Drugs

Dependency on drugs is another aspect of life-style worth examining. Although we are being educated to the adverse effects of drugs, we as a society continue to use them. Whether it is an addiction requiring an increase on a daily basis or a social addiction, it, too, like smoking and drinking, offers no benefit to the human body.

The use of drugs during pregnancy is being studied constantly. Women who take drugs when they are pregnant are more likely to deliver premature babies with a low birth weight. Addiction to drugs means an increase in need and frequency. It is draining financially and may result in desperate behavior.

Cocaine, for example, is a vasoconstricting drug. That means it cuts down the free flow of blood through the vessels. For a pregnant woman, that means the uterus and placenta do not receive an adequate blood flow. The baby is not being properly nourished by the placenta, and its growth is stunted. The baby is smaller than normal and may be intolerant of the labor. His start on life is compromised by his mother's dependence on drugs.

The hope is that most woman find pregnancy a time for new beginnings. Habits like smoking, drinking, and drugs may require serious help. Mental health centers or hospitals with specific drug rehabilitation programs are available to counsel and help with drug and alcohol dependency. It may even mean admission to a detoxification center and full-time help of professionals.

A life free from harmful habits is a life ready to consider pregnancy. It is said that old habits are hard to break but not impossible. Believe you can, and seek help from others.

### Smoking

Studies show that cigarette smoking is linked to 25 percent of all cancer deaths in women. Smoking also affects fertility: it can actually increase the time it takes to conceive. Fertilization, implantation, and development of the egg can be significantly affected by smoking.

Not only is conception influenced but the welfare of the baby is as well. Fetal growth retardation is a condition that affects the growing fetus. The baby's length, weight, and body mass are all affected. Smoking causes hypoxia, or a decrease in the oxygen going to the placenta and uterus. Both are the life source for the baby.

The smoker considering pregnancy should evaluate her diet before conceiving. Women who smoke quite often do so for weight control. They feel if they smoke a cigarette, they can satisfy hunger urges and avoid weight gain. While this may be the case, it also promotes a poor diet. Women considering pregnancy may need to develop new eating habits that will meet nutritional demands. This will be an area of special concentration to build up your body and release it from cigarettes forever.

Understanding *why* you smoke is the first step to fighting the urge. Some people smoke to relieve tension, cravings, or anxieties. Some receive positive feelings from smoking. Other people just do it out of habit, without rhyme or reason.

You should also try to understand *when* you smoke. Some people smoke before meals or afterward. Others do it when they are talking on the telephone, driving, reading, writing, or in the presence of another smoker.

One of the first things to do to help yourself stop is to monitor yourself. Notice the times of the day and what you are doing that cues you to smoke. Keep a written journal of this information. Your next step includes modifying your life-style so that you can begin to quit.

Groups like the American Heart Association and the American Cancer Society offer programs to help people stop smoking. Help can be sought through counseling, hypnosis, acupuncture, and other means.

### Chemicals and Additives

Growing a garden or owning a farm may be the only way to avoid chemicals in food. Unless your fruits and vegetables have been hand-sown and harvested, there is no guarantee that they were not exposed to chemicals like pesticides. Animal products such as beef, fish, and poultry are also heavily influenced by the chemical world. Beef and poultry are treated with growth hormones and antibiotics. Fish are raised on farms or fall victim to water pollution like mercury poisoning.

Additives are in every food found in cans, boxes, meats, and little envelopes for dieters. Saccharine, nitrates, and artificial colors are just a few to be avoided.

Artificial sweeteners are still being questioned as to their role in cancer and birth defects. Artificial colorings have been found to influence the hyperactivity of children. Nitrates and nitrites fill our hot dogs, salami, and other cured meats. It makes one wonder what they were curing it of?

What can we do to rise above this discouraging news about the food we are so dependent on? Here are a few ideas:

- Read labels and study what foods are chemical culprits.
- If you buy fresh vegetables and fruits, scrub them before eating. Use warm soapy water. Even in the grocery store, some of the fresh produce is "dressed up" to be more appealing.
- Have a farmer raise a steer for you. Some farmers will do this for a fee. Sometimes they will offer a half or quarter of a steer for sale. Just make sure that the farmer is not adding hormones or chemicals to the feed. The usual arrangement includes the cost of the calf, its feed, other maintenance costs, and the charge for butchering and wrapping the meat.
- Seafoods that are the safest are from the ocean. Tuna, sea bass,

cod, halibut, sole, flounder, and snapper are preferred.
- Try to cook from scratch. You will stand a better chance of receiving nutritious ingredients.
- Develop eating habits aimed at recognizing what is potentially toxic to you and your baby.
- Consider drinking spring water. Bottled water can be purchased by the case. Well water and city water supplies can be potential sources of contamination. Have your water tested frequently if you are using a well.

## COMMON CENTS EATING

Buying food is a major financial investment. Establishment of a healthy diet does not necessarily mean an increase in your grocery bill. Consumers are influenced by TV commercials, magazines, and the ever-promising coupons. Food manufacturers must convince you that their product is the best, and worth the cost, no matter what.

The good news is that the highly competitive food industry creates healthy competition and more choices for the consumer. Comparative shopping is an especially important skill to learn. By law, the contents of each product must be listed on the label or wrapper. Comparing brand "A" and brand "B" for content, quality, and price is what comparative shopping is all about.

Different stores will have different prices for the same food. Convenience stores have an increase in retail price of at least 40 to 50 percent. If at all possible, shop in a grocery store. A large grocery store will run advertisements in the newspaper. If you do not want to put in the leg work of traveling from one store to another for comparative shopping, read the paper. If you are looking for an item not listed in the paper, call around for comparative prices.

Common cents eating requires only a few basic principles. A change in eating habits may mean a change in buying food as well. Try these ideas for a "cents-able" change:
- Fresh is best. Buy fresh fruits, vegetables, and meat. Summer is an excellent time to stock up on fresh produce. Freezing is an effective way to store it without total loss of essential vitamins and nutrients.
- Cheap meats are hard to beat. Poultry and seafood are still your best bet for economical and healthy meat sources. They are high in protein with a low cholesterol content.
- Read that label. American consumers are reading labels as a matter

33

of preservation. The order in which the contents appear will tell you which ingredient is predominant.

- What is in a name? The brand name plays an important role in how much you spend or save in the grocery store. There may be a need to compromise to get the same nutritional value at a lower cost. For example, a coupon for Cheerios might discount the price by 20 cents. If you do not eat Cheerios and prefer Oatsies, 80 cents less than the Cheerios, then the coupon is really worthless. If the content is the same, why not save a few cents and forget the highly advertised name?

- Shopping is a lifetime skill. At first, comparative shopping may seem to take longer. Reading labels may seem like a big waste of time to some shoppers. You will have the last laugh when you and your co-shopper approach the checkout counter. While you can pay cash for your groceries, she will be making financial arrangements with the manager. It is worth the time to save a buck.

## SUGGESTED READING

*As You Eat So Your Baby Grows*
Nikki Goldbeck
Ceres Press, 1977

*Nourishing Your Unborn Child*
Phyllis Williams
Avon Books, 1982

*The Dieter's Dilemma: Eating Less and Weighing More*
William Bennett and Joel Gurin
Basic Books, Inc., 1982

*Eating for the Eighties: A Complete Guide to Vegetarian Nutrition*
Jamie Coulter Harbarger and Neil Hartbarger
Saunders Press, 1981

*A Woman's Conflict:*
*The Special Relationship Between Women and Food*
Jane Rachel Kaplan
Prentice-Hall, 1980

*Community Food Education Handbook*
Ellen Weiss, Harriet Davidson,
Laurie Heise, and Nance Petit
Agricultural Marketing Project, 1980
Distributed by the
Cooperative Food Education Program
2606 Westwood Drive
Nashville, TN 37204
Copyright 1980 by
Agricultural Marketing Project

*The Obsession:*
*Reflections on the Tyranny of Slenderness*
Kim Chernin
Harper and Row, 1981

*Nutrition for Your Pregnancy*
The University of Minnesota Guide
Judith Brown
University of Minnesota Press,
Minneapolis, Minn.

*How to be Your Own Nutritionist*
Stuart M. Berger, M.D.
Avon Books, 1987

*Cut Your Grocery Bills in Half*
Barbara Salsbury with Cheri Loveless
Acropolis Books, Ltd., 1983

*Beat the Supermarket Blues and*
*Eat Well, Too!*
Marsha Giles and Joyce Convay
Purpose Books, 1984

*It's All on the Label:*
*Understanding Food, Additives, and Nutrition*
Zenas Block
Little, Brown and Company, 1981

35

## RESOURCE GROUPS

Food and Nutrition Information Center
National Agriculture Library Building
Room 304
Beltsville, MD 20705
301-344-3719
Information on nutrition

*The Consumer Information Catalog*
Consumer Information Center
Pueblo, CO 81009
This catalog is available free from the center. It contains information on children, food, nutrition, health, exercise, and weight control.

*American Anorexia Bulimia Association, Inc.*
133 Cedar Lane
Teaneck, NJ 07666
201-836-1800

*Weight Watchers International*
Jericho Atrium
500 N. Broadway
Jericho, NY 11753-2196
516-939-0400

*The National Association For Gardening*
180 Flynn Avenue
Burlington, VT 05401
Publishes newsletter and other literature.

*National Nutrition Education Clearing House*
Society for Nutrition Education
2140 Shattuck Avenue, Suite 1110
Berkeley, CA 94704
415-548-1363
Printed audiovisual material available in English and Spanish, for lay and professional persons.

National Clearinghouse for Alcoholic Information
Box 2345
Rockville, MD 20852
301-468-2600

National Clearinghouse for Drug Abuse Information
P.O. Box 416
Kensington, MD 20795
301-468-2600

CHAPTER 4

# PHYSICAL CONDITIONING
## Shaping Up for the Future

*"It is the nature of a man as he grows older. . .to protest against change, particularly change for the better."*
—John Steinbeck

## DOWN TO BASICS

Each spring, farmers stand and survey their fields anticipating the crops that will burst forth from the ground. They have worked the ground and revived it after a long, cold winter. Preparation for planting the seeds that will bear the fruit of their labors is not taken lightly. It is their business to nurture and cultivate fields and harvest crops to feed the world.

The same conscious efforts to prepare so carefully should be made by women considering pregnancy. First she can examine what she has to work with. The body of a woman is unique in that it can create, with the sperm of a man, a human life. Just as the farmer realizes the potential of his fields, women must understand that the possibilities are endless in creating the best environment in which a baby will grow.

Physical fitness has many dimensions. Internal fitness, influenced by nutrition or lack of it, is as vital as the sun and rain are to the earth. External fitness is more than just building muscles and looking good on the beach. Conditioning becomes more practical to the woman thinking about conception.

Carrying a child during pregnancy is demanding on different body systems. Zeroing in on specific areas for conditioning will help increase endurance for pregnancy, labor, and delivery as well as promote a rapid recovery.

## OUTSIDE CONDITIONING: WHAT IS ALL THE FUSS?

It is estimated that 15 to 20 million women in the United States are active participants in some type of exercise program. Working women, mothers at home, teenagers, and retired women are realizing that it is never too soon or too late to develop a physical conditioning regime.

The body is a complex system of checks and balances. Muscles, nerves, bones, and a variety of vessels run this machine, like parts in a car. If one area is not pulling its share of the work, other areas also suffer. Establishment of a conditioning program before conception is the ideal approach.

It is believed that development of muscle strength, flexibility, and endurance can make pregnancy and delivery easier. Research has been conducted on women who maintained a physical conditioning program throughout pregnancy. They found the rate of cesarean section births lower, the babies' birth weights higher, the hospital stays shorter, and the women's self-image improved.

## How to Begin

Developing an exercise program involves a few serious considerations. First, the program should be aimed at developing flexibility, strength, and endurance. Next, it should be done on a regular basis. Third, it should include a warm-up and a cool-down period. That is why it is important to develop a program custom-made for you. The time, place, and frequency of your exercise must fit into your life. It is important to be realistic about conditioning goals.

There are a variety of exercises available for conditioning. Women with a particular sport interest can add exercises to their sporting program to achieve complete conditioning. For example, walking is great for muscle strength and improving circulation. What it cannot do is build endurance. Either jogging or biking is good for endurance building, but neither do anything for the arms. That brings us to swimming, considered one of the best forms of exercise. It uses muscles and develops flexibility and cardiovascular and respiratory endurance. If you live close to a pool and can swim, this may be the conditioner for you.

Some women enjoy group exercise programs or sports. The group motivation and support may be the nudge some women need to get started. Others prefer the privacy of their homes with Jane Fonda on the VCR.

If your partner is in need of conditioning, now is the time for him to become involved. Some couples find working together on diets and exercise programs helpful. Other couples may find this disastrous. The important factor is to be consistent and disciplined in the amount of time invested.

Whether you want to invest in leotards and shimmery tights or basic gray sweats, make sure you are comfortable. High cotton content and an open weave for evaporation of sweat are two important qualities in exercise clothing.

A good supportive bra is imperative. Special sports bras are available. For preservation and support of breast tissue, and to prevent injury, be sure to invest in good breast support.

Shoes should fit properly and be supportive to the arch. Sporting goods stores and fitness specialty shops have trained personnel who can help you choose the best shoe for your activity and your pocketbook.

From head to toe, fashionable or frumpy, be comfortable and supportive of your body.

## Let's Go

The clothes have been chosen, a disciplined attitude is established, and the time to do it has been set aside. So what is available for you? There are exercises to condition every part of the body. More important, they need to be performed properly to be beneficial. For example, jumping jacks are great for endurance, but if your elbows are bent and your arms never reach above your shoulders, then the stretching of arms and trunk is lost. Quality versus quantity is a vital concept to successful workouts.

Each exercise session should begin with a warm-up period of about five to ten minutes. This is done for several reasons:

1. It prevents sudden stress to the body.

2. It increases the blood flow to the muscles, making them more responsive to a workout.

3. With an increase in flexibility, there will be less chance of injury.

The exercise session should last at least 30 minutes and be followed by a ten-minute cool-down. Make it a gradual process, allowing your body to stretch out and cool down.

## Key Body Parts for Pregnancy

Specific areas of the preconceptional woman's body should be conditioned. The pregnant body changes almost without notice by the mother-to-be. The growing uterus slowly enlarges, moves out of the pelvic cavity, and begins to push the other organs aside. Perhaps the area receiving the greatest stress is the back.

"Stand up straight!" is the order heard most by the growing teenager, and the one least carried out. Good posture means that the muscles and the spine are in alignment while standing upright. The muscles of the back, back of hips, front of the thigh, and back of the legs are fighting the force of gravity. No wonder that by the end of the day, our shoulders meet in the middle, and our poor bodies are practically bent in half. Poorly developed muscles in the hip and abdominal areas quite often lead to improper posture.

The Erector Spinae group of muscles runs along both sides of the spinal column. Weakness in these muscles, especially in the lower back, increases the curvature, leading to strain on the spinal discs in the spinal column. As the growing uterus is pulling these muscles forward, the chance of developing a lower backache on a daily basis is increased.

The Rectus Abdominus group of muscles starts at the fifth, sixth, and seventh ribs and goes to the pubic bone. These muscles, properly toned, can produce that appealing flat abdomen. Pregnancy divides and separates the rectus muscles as the uterus rises out of the pelvic cavity. Developing strength in this area will be beneficial for several reasons:

1. The strength and flexibility of abdominal muscles will allow for elasticity.

2. Strong abdominal muscles will support the enlarging uterus.

3. Strength from these conditioned muscles will allow the woman in labor to be more effective during the final stage of delivery, when she must push the baby out.

The thighs and buttocks will benefit from conditioning. These muscles include gluteals and the quadriceps femoris. These muscle groups need to be strengthened and stretched. They are pulling against gravity constantly.

With the additional weight of pregnancy, and the shift of the center of balance, the stress is increased. Many women may find they waddle while they are pregnant. This is due to weakened lower back, buttock, and thigh muscles. Keep in mind that conditioning before pregnancy will prevent or lessen many of the discomforts women experience in the last few months of pregnancy.

The upper body, chest muscles, and arms are not to be neglected. Among the weakest areas of the average woman are her pectoral, or chest, muscles. During pregnancy, the breasts increase in weight as much as one-half pound per breast. Some will say that the best thing about being pregnant is that finally there is some cleavage. The fact remains that strong chest muscles will be additional support for the growing breasts.

The breasts are preparing themselves for nourishment of the baby.

Contrary to popular belief, breast-feeding does not cause sagging breasts. It is still the best food for your baby and is an experience like no other. We use our arms daily as women on the go, and yet their development is not actively pursued. Upper arm and forearm muscles need to be conditioned as well. The triceps and biceps muscles are challenged with the occurrence of motherhood. If you have ever rocked or carried a baby for hours on end, you know that your arms begin to give out after the first half hour. Pushing a stroller and carrying a diaper bag while shopping not only builds your coordination but your arms as well.

A conditioning program for a concerned woman would not be complete without Kegel exercises, which are extremely beneficial. These exercises are designed for those muscles that cannot be seen, but nevertheless need to be toned. The pelvic floor muscles form a figure eight around the urinary, vaginal, and rectal openings. This area needs to be strengthened for its role in childbirth as well as for other benefits.

The first step for most women is to identify the muscles. The best way to do this is to sit on the toilet and begin to urinate. Once the stream has started, stop it. On occasion, we have all been called away from the bathroom by a ringing telephone. We will either push or stop our flow of urine and pull up our pants and fly to the phone. The credit for either of those talents goes to the perineal muscles. Starting and stopping the flow of urine is just one way to recognize the location of these muscles. Advantages of performing Kegels are as follows:

- They increase the blood circulation to the area, which promotes healing and elasticity following childbirth or surgery.
- With regular exercise, the woman may be able to recognize the muscles and learn to relax them at the time of delivery.
- There may even be avoidance of a prolapsed uterus (when the uterus begins to drop out of its location inside the abdomen and protrude into the vagina) or avoidance of a cystocele (when the bladder protrudes into the vagina). Both conditions result from weakened tissues and muscles, causing the uterus and bladder to actually move downward.
- These exercises have been known to increase bladder control and help avoid stress incontinence, which is the leakage of urine when a person coughs, sneezes, laughs, or strains.
- The best is kept until last. Kegel exercises can enhance sexual pleasure for a woman and her lover. It is indeed a pleasure to practice on your partner.

43

How do you do Kegel exercises? Anywhere, anytime, and in any position. Assume a comfortable position either sitting, standing, or lying down. First, contract and hold the muscle for the count of three. Next, release and relax. The exercise is repeated 6 to 10 times per session. These toning techniques may be performed 50 to 60 times a day. Remember, any muscle can suffer from fatigue, so don't overdo it.

## SPORTS

There are only a few sports in which women do not participate. The barriers have been broken, so jockeys, basketball players, and downhill skiers are no longer only men. Women golf, swim, ice skate and roller skate, fence, jog, run, and play most games that include a ball. There are pregnant golfers and great Olympic runners who are thirty-year-old mothers.

Women athletes have been studied, especially once they have decided to become moms. It has been proven that they not only have normal pregnancies but also quite often have shorter labor and delivery times. They are health-conscious, well-tuned, muscle-toned women. They understand how their bodies work and what they can tolerate.

In fact, active women have fewer complications in pregnancy. They experience less toxemia, fewer backaches, and fewer premature deliveries. They also have about half of the chance of having a cesarean section birth compared with inactive women.

While it is not necessary to become a world-class athlete, any activity that gets you moving can only be of benefit. A sporting activity in addition to an exercise program is a winning combination. If you have any medical condition that prohibits active sports participation, consult your doctor to help you choose the best exercise program for you.

What is available for the novice athlete? Anything you want, can afford, and can fit into your life-style. Here are a few favorites enjoyed by women.

### Swimming

This sport is at the top of the list as a complete activity for the preconceptional, pregnant, and postpartum woman ready to tone up her body. It builds stamina, increases cardiopulmonary (heart and lungs) fitness, and increases flexibility and strength. It works every muscle system, especially the upper body, which is a weak area for women.

The benefit of buoyancy in the water is great for anyone who is over-weight. It is perfect for the pregnant woman. This is one of the few sports that is complete in the benefits it offers. You must have access to a pool and be willing to swim on a regular basis.

## Bicycling

The basic equipment would include a bike, mobile or stationary, a hel-met for street riding, and a good pair of shoes. Biking requires coordina-tion and stamina. As with any sport, begin slowly and work up the endurance ladder. The legs and cardiopulmonary system receive the most benefit from biking.

The stationary bike may be more practical if the great outdoors is not at your disposal. At times, it may be safer to be indoors instead of in rush hour traffic. Once pregnancy occurs, you will need to be aware of the shift in your center of gravity. With that adjustment in mind, your biking days can continue.

## Golf

Unless you live in southern California or Florida, the practicality of golf may depend on Mother Nature. In general, it is a sport that strengthens the upper body and requires flexibility and trunk strength. Endurance to walk the three-mile hike of an eighteen-hole course is also good for the cardiovascular system.

## Jogging or Running

These sports are both easy to do and inexpensive. They will require investing in a good supportive pair of shoes. Basic coordination, flexi-bility, and endurance add to the enjoyment of these sports. Neither is a complete sport in the sense that the repetition of the activity does not develop other areas of the body.

It is important to keep in mind basic thermal rules. Keep warm when running in the winter, and keep cool in the summer. If you decide to continue to run after you conceive, wear a support bra for your growing breasts, and be sure not to overheat.

Your body is undergoing hormonal shifts and what used to be a cas-ual run may make you feel faint or pass out. If you decide to continue to jog after conceiving, be sure to discuss it with your doctor or midwife.

## Tennis

This is another sport that takes the whole body into consideration for conditioning. It can increase endurance if played often and hard enough. It requires flexibility and some upper body strength of the arms and wrists. The legs and back also benefit from this popular sport. Once pregnancy occurs, consider the shift in your center of gravity. If you are unsure of the safety of playing while in late pregnancy, contact your care giver.

## Walking

This is the sport of all ages, all physical conditions, and all occupations. Everyone can walk for exercise. While it is not an endurance-building activity and it does not strengthen any special muscle group, it is refreshing. It is excellent for the circulation and for the respiratory system.

The woman who is pregnant may need to rely on walking for her form of sport. It is readily available for the low, low price of time.

Invest in a supportive pair of shoes to avoid leg and foot problems. Make an attempt to maintain good posture and proper body alignment while walking.

## Other Sports

Any activity involving contact with other players, for example, volleyball, softball, basketball, and soccer, should be eliminated as pregnancy progresses. Gymnastics requires balance and coordination, both of which are compromised as pregnancy advances.

Horseback riding develops excellent leg muscles, balance, and coordination. It is not, however, a practical sport to count on to continue throughout your pregnancy.

While many sports seem to give the body a complete workout, there is still a need for exercises to enhance any sport. Even something as minor as being a right-handed tennis player leaves the athlete with a weaker left arm. Combining a sport, an exercise program, and healthy food intake will strengthen and condition your body.

Based on a body weight of 125 pounds, the following sporting activities burn calories on an hourly basis as follows:

Bicycling 5.5 mph—251
Archery—268
Golf with two players—271

Ping-Pong—194
Rowing machine—684
Climbing a hill—488
Running 5.5 mph—537
Skiing downhill—483
Swimming
  Backstroke—194
  Butterfly—586
  Side stroke—418
Tennis—347

It is important to be able to fit any sport, exercise program, and diet into your life and continue to follow through with it. This is not to say that you should not try a different combination from time to time. That is okay. In fact, things could get boring if at some point you did not try another challenging sport.

Daily living activities have calorie-burning benefits as well. The following activities are based on calories burned per hour. It may be difficult to perform some of these activities for an hour or more, but it is welcome news that you can burn calories and accomplish tasks at the same time:

Cleaning windows—207
Dancing—209
Talking—92
Mopping—227
Office work—150
Driving—150
Weeding the garden—295
Eating—70
Making the bed—196
Shoveling snow—389
Walking 2 mph—176
Walking upstairs—869
Walking downstairs—333
Watching TV—60

An active life releases tension, increases energy, and helps boost self-esteem. It is something you can choose for yourself and fit into your unique life-style. A sport or exercise program or both will benefit you now and forever. Claim a healthy living program for you and your baby.

## MAKING A CHOICE: WHAT IS RIGHT FOR YOU?

With all the options examined, the choice is up to you. Deciding on an exercise program, a sport, and nutritional and diet changes is your next move. The most important consideration to keep in mind is that what you choose works for you. It is not enough to begin living a healthy, well-thought-out life and let it go by the wayside after conception and birth. Following through is vital for a lifetime of healthy living for you, your mate, and your child.

Your care giver will be able to help you decide how much weight you should lose and at what point he would recommend it safe to consider conceiving. As was already noted, while you are dieting is not a safe time to attempt to get pregnant and could be harmful to you and your baby.

Study the exercises available and decide which areas of your body you want to improve. Take into consideration that with the enlargement of your uterus during pregnancy, you may not be able to follow through with some of the exercises you are performing now. You may find it necessary to modify them in order to protect yourself from injury.

The improvement of eating habits is probably the greatest change you will make. Knowing what influence good foods have on your body and what it takes to create a child, you will find improved eating habits to benefit you both.

Becoming food conscious is a lifetime skill. There is no need to hold a degree in dietary science to understand what your body needs. It is a basic theory of supplying what is essential for life and avoiding that which destroys life. Chemicals, additives, alcohol, and caffeine are just a few of the enemies of your diet.

Now it is up to you. Choose healthy eating habits, a consistent exercise program, a care giver to work with you, and an attitude of wanting the best for you and your baby. If it works for you, then it is the perfect choice.

## SUGGESTED READING

*The Sports Doctors Fitness Book for Women*
John Marshall, M.D., and Heather Barbash
Delacorte, 1981

*Every Woman's Health*
Eighteen Women Doctors
Doubleday, 1985

*Suzy Prudden's Spot Reducing Program*
Suzy Prudden and Jeffrey Sussman
Workman, 1979

*Essential Exercises for the Childbearing Year*
Elizabeth Noble
Houghton Mifflin, 1982

*Sports for Life*
Robert Buxbaum and Lyle J. Micheli
Beacon Press, 1979

## RESOURCE GROUPS

National Women's Health Network
224 Seventh Street, S.E.
Washington, D.C. 20003
202-347-1140

American Heart Association
7320 Greenville Avenue
Dallas, TX 75231
214-373-6300

The National Foundation for the March of Dimes
1275 Mamoroneck Avenue
White Plains, NY 10605
914-428-7100
Information concerning the importance of a healthy pregnancy for a
healthy baby.

Sportsline
1-800-227-3988
415-536-6266 (Alaska, Hawaii, and California)
Information for women on sports, physical fitness, and sports machines.

CHAPTER 5

# CHANGES AND CHALLENGES OF THE HEAD

*"The greatest revolution of our generation is the discovery that human beings, by changing the inner attitudes of their minds can change the outer aspects of their lives."*

—William James

## WHY START NOW?

"Let's have a baby. They are so cute and lovable. Life would be so nice with a baby in our home. How about it, Roger?" Dana queried.

"Sure, Dana, give me five good reasons for having a baby." Dana was left speechless. While she was indeed able to come up with at least five reasons, which ones were sensible?

While couples are realizing the importance of preconceptional planning, they may be overlooking the whys of having a baby. Exploring some possible reasons will enable the preconceptional couple to focus on their own motivation.

Everyone at some point realizes that he or she is mortal. Having a child will enable a piece of each parent to live on for another generation. Carrying on the family name is a very strong desire in some families. It would be a tragedy for the family who is depending on this if all the kids are girls who will marry and change their names.

Women who are not being true to themselves may seek conception to keep their husband or partner close. Repairing a troubled marriage should be done before conception. It is an unfortunate truth that the birth of a child will not mend already tense relationships.

For some women, the birth of a child signifies passage into adulthood. It is viewed by society as a positive transition. What is overlooked is that a woman may base her total self-worth on becoming a mother. When her last child is grown and ready to leave home, she may feel as if she no longer has a purpose. Without the development of outside interests or a circle of friends, she is left feeling empty.

Well-meaning families can put pressure on couples to reproduce. Usually the newlyweds are safe for about a year before they begin to receive the sometimes not-so-subtle hints. "When are we going to see some grandchildren? Your brothers and sisters have children, how about you kids? You are not getting any younger. You might not be able to have any if you wait any longer."

If family pressure is not enough, how about peer pressure? Sometimes friends with kids begin to seek friendships with others in the same familial situation. The childless couple may feel excluded. They may be encouraged, almost pushed by their friends into making the move. Is it because the friends are truly convinced that there is nothing on earth like parenting, or do they want you to be in the same boat? Whatever reasons friends give for wanting their childless friends to conceive, it is just another form of peer pressure. It is as if they are putting the heat on about having sex for the first time. This time they do not want you to use a condom. Beware of peers and their stories of pain-free labor and days of blissful parenting.

Just when women thought things were looking up in the career world, they started hearing the tick of the ever-present biological clock. Women have fought through barriers keeping them from equal opportunities for years. The one area of life women have no real control over is the time allotted for conception.

The biological clock begins ticking in each woman from the day she receives her first period. The average age for this occurrence is around 12 years old. Women remain fertile typically into their early forties. It is in this thirty-year period that women are given the opportunity to reproduce. If there are no fertility problems or other prohibiting medical problems, most women will conceive.

Today, women are purposely delaying childbirth. What is happening is that although women are waiting before starting a family, the clock continues to tick. This means that pressure from our own bodies to produce in a limited time then influences when conception occurs. The age of the woman may also determine how easily she can become pregnant (see chap. 13). It is a good idea to discuss with your partner why now is the time to consider having a baby.

## FREEDOM IS JUST ANOTHER WORD FOR CHILDLESS

What will it be like to go from a twosome to a trio? It could be quite a transition if the couple is not prepared. Parenting is one of those jobs that requires on-the-job training. It may be of some help to do some baby-sitting. If friends or family members have a newborn or toddler, ask them to loan their children to you for several hours. While it is a fact that everyone else's children will be different from your own, it gives you a good idea of what parenting may involve.

The physical demands of pregnancy may have an effect on the couple's life-style. Women are choosing to work up to the day they deliver their babies. They may be forced to financially, or they may choose to keep busy. Whatever the reason, it is not unusual to see women pack their briefcase and suitcase during their last few weeks of pregnancy. This may be the plan, but the baby may have another.

Donna and Bill decided to have a baby. Donna was a well-organized nurse, and Bill was an independent contractor. Because Bill did most of his work outside during the summer, Donna calculated the best time for the birth would be in the winter. This way Bill could watch the baby after she returned to work. Donna had planned on using her six-week maternity leave. It seemed like a well-thought-out strategy.

What Donna did not count on was morning sickness. Not only was it morning sickness but it was around the clock. She suffered from hyperemesis, a condition causing her to vomit constantly. She had to be hospitalized for several weeks. She was given intravenous fluids and medications to help her stop vomiting. This was not part of her plan. Needless to say, she was very discouraged.

Donna's condition lasted several months. She was able to maintain the pregnancy and deliver a healthy baby girl. After what seemed like an impossible start, Donna and Bill were able to adapt to parenthood.

The physical demands of pregnancy are different for each person. Allowing for the unexpected will make this change easier to handle.

The role change from adult to parent can be quite a transition. It is as if something magical occurs on the birth of a child. It is one of the miracles of life, this is true. What it does not mean is that parenthood is zapped into the bodies and minds of the baby producers.

It is usually after the pregnancy is known that the experts emerge. People tend to relate every tragic pregnancy and birth experience they can possibly remember to the newly pregnant woman. Why? Do they want to heighten her anxiety just a little more? Is it necessary to relate the story of the woman who labored for three days and nights? Did these stories really happen, or are they from a supermarket tabloid?

These pressures from outside sources possess little benefit. The pregnant couple must try to establish their own thoughts on pregnancy.

They should understand that theirs is unique from any other pregnancy. Their child will be totally different from other children, because they are the parents.

The pregnant woman many feel the outside influence more often than the father-to-be. After all, she has been preceded by her own mother and mother-in-law. What will she be able to handle, if she can at all? More often than not, a woman will doubt her skills as a mother before a man doubts his ability to father. Mutual support is important at this time. Believing in each other and your skills as parents should begin before the baby arrives.

The baby is here, and the parenting experience is going well. So why are the new parents so unhappy? Could it be because they cannot just take off to the shore for the weekend anymore? Could it be because they cannot stay out all night with their friends, especially since she is breast-feeding? The sense of being held prisoner in a house with a baby is a common feeling.

It is all right to feel this way. If the couple understands long before the baby comes that there is a temporary time of adjustment, they will survive. Like any new job, in the beginning, it takes time to become comfortable and proficient. At times, it seems like you will never get the hang of it. But as you have proven to yourself before, you do become comfortable and even enjoy it.

Dale and Becky enjoyed their weekly poker game with their friends. They liked to entertain, so it was no problem to hold the game at their house each week. What they did not realize was how different their lives could be after they had their first child, Katy.

Dale saw no reason that they should not continue to host poker games even after they had the baby. It did occur to Becky that nursing a new baby every three hours and suffering from sleep deprivation made her feel somewhat resentful and overwhelmed. Not only could she not enjoy a beer with the game but she had to keep jumping up to see if Katy was crying. Her jitteriness, not uncommon to new mothers, was not noticed by her friends, who had no children.

Becky had finally had enough when someone asked, "Hey, Becky, is that a baby crying?" She threw her cards in the air and stormed out of the room in tears. It was then that Dale realized what was happening. He asked their friends to leave and said that he would call them sometime.

As new parents, it is not possible to realize exactly what roles you can continue to play. Like Becky and Dale, couples may believe that it is no big deal to entertain and parent a newborn at the same time. Friends and family are not always sensitive to what adjustments you need to make.

Moving from being a couple to being a family is a major transition and most certainly a change in life-style. Acceptance of this change will make the transition easier for you as a couple. True friends will understand and support your need to be alone as a new family. Assert yourself, but gently. It is a wonderful thing to have friends who can then become your child's friends as well.

## SETTING LIMITS

While setting limits with friends may be uncomfortable, dealing with intrusive family members may seem impossible. Involvement of family members like parents, siblings, aunts, uncles, and even your grandparents is important.

Our society has gotten away from family closeness and camaraderie. We are highly mobile. Corporations relocate families at a moment's notice, taking them away from supportive families and friends.

There are both advantages and disadvantages to living near our extended families.

### Advantages:

1. Support: This is found in emotional, physical, and sometimes financial support.

2. Network for the Child: A child with a supportive extended family has a multitude of family members to call on for different needs.

3. Guidance: Because families may tend to share similar rearing beliefs, the child receives consistent guidance.

### Disadvantages:

1. Closeness vs. Interference: Living close to relatives can lead to a tendency for everyone to give their opinion on the child's care and discipline, perhaps confusing the child.

2. Support vs. Challenge: What may start out as helpful support can turn into a challenge of your parenting choices.

3. Financial Support: In accepting financial support, relatives may feel they have an investment and say in your family decisions.

Setting limits with family members may be a new experience. It includes learning to be assertive and not being afraid to risk stepping on toes if necessary. There is a difference, however, between assertiveness and aggression. One will benefit you, the other will not.

We tend to deal with situations in one of three ways. We remain silent and put our own feelings behind, wanting to avoid conflict. We can explode when pushed and risk violating the rights of other people for our own beliefs. Or, we can think the situation through and find a middle-of-the-road solution, without totally giving up our wishes. That is being assertive.

Assertiveness is a healthy skill to acquire for all aspects of life but especially during pregnancy and child rearing. Pregnancy is a time when women want to be taught all they can learn and do whatever it takes to assure a healthy baby. Along with that comes an undying trust in the experts. This could be doctor, midwife, mother, sister, or experienced friend. While you are grateful for advice, you need to choose what is right for you.

Mary and Al were excited about their pregnancy and willing to do everything their doctor told them to do. Because Mary was 38 years old, her doctor told her he wanted to perform an amniocentesis. This test of the amniotic fluid in the uterus would detect the presence of Down's Syndrome. The test possessed risks for the baby, and if there were problems, Mary could have a miscarriage. The doctor suggested that if the test were positive for Down's, Mary should have a therapeutic abortion and try to get pregnant again.

It was a difficult decision, but Mary and Al decided against the test. They had tried so long to get pregnant, and both knew it was not realistic for them to keep trying. Having made their decision, they discussed it with their doctor. He argued against their decision. Mary and Al, realizing that they knew what was best for them, stood by their decision not to have the test. They wanted this baby, just the way it was. Six months later, a healthy baby boy was placed in Mary's arms. They had made a choice and asserted themselves accordingly.

This is not to say that it is always necessary to doubt or challenge your care giver's advice. It is a good idea to have all your questions answered concerning testing and procedures for yourself and your baby. Learning to be assertive before pregnancy will allow you to feel secure in the decisions you make.

Family members may need to be dealt with in an assertive manner. They may feel strongly about beliefs concerning pregnancy and parenthood. Mothers and mothers-in-law may have more experience than you, but that does not necessarily mean it is right for you.

Fathers and fathers-in-law are not exempt from giving advice. Parents never really stop parenting, but what they view as helpful advice may feel like interference. Allow them to express their thoughts, try to be considerate, but at the same time, feel secure in your own selves to express your personal preferences and choices.

## BODY CHANGES

Pregnancy means adjustment to a body that undergoes changes and challenges. Conception signals the woman's hormones to create a body that will house, nourish, and deliver a baby.

In the first few months, the pregnant woman may react more emotionally than she usually does. Some women do not seem to notice many changes, others feel like crying constantly. Ambivalence toward the pregnancy can confuse a woman. She knows she is happy to be pregnant, and yet she is saddened. This is a perfectly normal symptom of pregnancy. Hormones play a part in this difficult period and will balance out in time.

This is a good time for women to express openly their concerns with their partners. Open communication is a necessity to put to rest some of the fears and concerns of pregnancy.

Pregnancy changes a woman's body forever. The conception and delivery of a baby changes your reproductive organs like the uterus, cervix, and breasts. The uterus changes by remaining somewhat larger than before you got pregnant, the cervix changes shape, and the breasts, having grown larger with breast milk, may seem different after pregnancy.

Our society is based on the physical appearance and attractiveness of our members. It is natural to strive to be slender and becoming. It is not typical that women want to be overweight. So how does pregnancy fit into our social standards?

Being pregnant is not a weight condition. Creating a life within a life is the most purposeful body change that can occur. The body changes that occur are influenced by the hormonal shift of pregnancy. The most obvious is the growing of the uterus. This organ is housed deep within the pelvic cavity and resembles a pear in size and shape. It houses, protects, and, with the help of the placenta, nourishes the baby. It grows upward and outward over a period of forty weeks. The uterus pushes other internal organs out of the way and stretches the muscles and skin of the abdomen.

Stretch marks may occur. Anyone who has ever lost a considerable amount of weight may experience stretch marks. Some women are concerned about the appearance of their skin after delivery. An excessive amount of weight gain will increase the likelihood of these marks. The skin is elastic enough to accommodate the growing abdomen and breasts without splitting open. It is not like a balloon, however, so that once you have delivered, it takes time for it to return to the prepregnant shape. This is not to say that time will erase stretch marks, necessarily.

With the understanding of why they occur and what they are, women can attempt to relieve their anxieties concerning both the emotional changes and physical changes of pregnancy.

## PREPARING FOR THE CHANGE

Realistic expectations of what parenthood will be like are important. What seems like the happiest time of life, the birth of a child, can be a nightmare. The demands placed on the couple or single mother can be overwhelming. Development of coping skills before conception will aid in a smooth transition into parenthood.

By definition, stress means a mentally or emotionally disruptive or disquieting influence. And while some people can handle it better than others, it can have a negative effect on pregnant women. Repeated exposure to stressful situations can cause a decrease in resistance to disease as well as the inability to utilize nutrients from the food we eat. Researchers have studied the effects of stress and anxiety during pregnancy. Rarely does a pregnant woman avoid worry about her baby's welfare, her own, or both.

Excessive concern creates fear and stress. This can lead to inner-body changes that cause a constriction of the blood vessels. These vessels can include those that feed the placenta and uterine muscles. Both can affect the baby, causing a decrease in the amount of oxygen the fetus receives.

Stress usually elicits a response from the people or person it affects. Stress is not the problem. How we cope with it is determined by our mental health. Stress is a part of normal living. Coping and maintaining equilibrium are what matters.

Some people deal with stress by having a good cry, sleeping, or withdrawing for a brief time. Our current social trends promote the use of drugs and alcohol to ease the pain. These means of coping are worthless. We are receiving the message that it is not good for us to be unhappy, and chemicals can help us.

We are each part of a human life cycle. We progress from birth, infancy, childhood, adolescence, young adulthood, middle age, to old age. There is stress within our life cycles. Because we are unique individuals, we experience stress from other sources as well.

For women experiencing motherhood, young adulthood means a time of establishment of self as an adult. Careers are being nurtured, relationships are being evaluated, and contemplation of the future is at hand. This stage of adulthood and the additional role of being a mother can be a stressful time.

Here are a few tips for coping with stress:

1. Change your position in relation to stress. For general coping, some people are able to move away from their source of stress. Babies are dependent on their parents for every part of their existence. You cannot run away from the parental role, nor would you want to. On occasion, if the stress becomes too great, and you feel there may be a danger to the child, call someone to come and give you a break.

A few hours away, by yourself, can do wonders for a stressed mother. Frustration and resentment are normal feelings for parents. When these feelings are recognized, it is easier to understand the need to be away. Make sure the baby is safe and taken care of and just walk away and regroup.

2. Gather information about the stress. Is the new baby noisy? Is he demanding at two o'clock in the morning? Does he insist on wetting his diapers? Does he seem to breast-feed for hours on end? If the answers are yes, it is because you have a typical healthy newborn.

These facts, when examined carefully, will help you realize that this is what new parents do for the first several weeks. The period of adjustment is like that of the honeymoon. Most people remember their honeymoon as being filled with warm thoughts and smiles. The real honeymoon began after you returned home. Then you found out what real life was like.

The new baby is like a third person moving in to stay. She has her ways of doing things, not meant to be irritating at all. She knows nothing more than her needs for food, comfort, love, and your company. Understanding the needs of a new baby may help decrease the stress of those first few weeks.

Taking the gathered information one step further may help the new mother identify some of her own feelings. Does the new mother feel inadequate as a mother, wife, lover, daughter, friend, executive, or employee? What you feel about yourself can influence the stress level. Carefully examine exactly where your feelings are coming from.

Is the new mother reacting to the baby, her spouse or lover, her lack of freedom, or to her physical state? Perhaps the leading cause of frustration among new mothers is sleep deprivation. This is a well-known phenomenon experienced by anyone only sleeping at two-hour intervals for days on end. Feelings of desperation and anxiety encompass the mother, making her feel crazy. Preparing for this may mean working out a plan preconceptionally with your partner.

At night, he may be the one who gets up with the baby to change and feed him. If the mother is breastfeeding, the father can change the baby and bring him to her. This way she can nurse in a relaxed manner. If there is a cradle in the room, she can then lay the baby down after nursing. Couples can cooperate to help each other through this time of change.

3. Have a flexible response to stress. The ability to gather information on the source of stress is best followed by a flexible response to stress. Now you know that you may be suffering from sleep deprivation. What else can you do to alleviate it? Sleep when baby sleeps. Have helpers through the day to perform housework and cook meals. This is particularly important if there are other children in the home.

Whatever the situation, the couple should attempt to develop a relaxed attitude. Anxiety only heightens when you try to resist the reality of the situation. With the information gained about what is realistic to expect from a new baby, the couple will be able to adjust and enjoy their new little bundle.

4. Redirect your energy. Energy is the one thing a new mother does not receive at her baby shower. In the first few weeks after the baby arrives, the new mother should rest and recover. If she has any athletic inclinations, she may begin to think about exercising. This is a healthy way of releasing stress and toning the body.

Some people create in order to release stress. Some enjoy making music, gardening, riding, jogging, biking, or swimming. This release is healthy and beneficial to both physical and mental health.

While the causes for the stress will not necessarily go away, exercise can clear the mind and improve self-esteem, both of which can benefit coping with stress. For any type of stress, talking with someone you trust is a form of therapy. Talking over problems is relating. This type of relationship is healthy and can be mutually supportive. Every person has her own way of coping. It is only when the skills do not work that there may be a need for professional guidance.

## Actively Handling Stress

There are other ways to handle stress and gain insight at the same time. The Eastern religions utilize yoga and other forms of meditation. Relaxation can be achieved by any number of methods. Below are a few of the more popular techniques.

### Yoga

This type of exercise works with the mind, body, and spirit. The word yoga means "union." There are basic aspects of yoga that include asanas, pranayama, and meditation.

Asanas are the physical postures used to stretch and relax the body. By focusing on these movements, the mind is able to push aside the concerns of the moment.

Pranayama are the breathing exercises used to increase the efficiency of respiration. Learning how to breathe properly will aid in relaxation of the body.

Meditation can be performed by anyone at any time. It is the conscious relaxation of the mind. It allows for the coming together of the physical, mental, and spiritual aspects.

Studies have proven that yoga possesses physical benefits. It is possible to lower blood pressure, increase joint flexibility, decrease the heart rate, improve hormonal function, and, of course, lower stress.

Meditation can be performed in any setting. It is performed for many different reasons. Some people like the calm feelings they experience. Others begin and end their day by meditation. It has its practical purposes, and yet it may go much deeper. Some people discover that they have an inner core. They find that they have needs to be met that are more than just physical. The spirit that enhances their life is recognized and responded to.

Meditation has been respected for centuries. Health practitioners have recognized the benefits and now encourage patients to participate in meditation. The potential benefits include the lowering of the heart rate, decrease in muscular tension, and the change in brain wave patterns, which creates a calm response to stress. This may aid in lowering the chances of heart attacks and strokes.

How to meditate is an individual preference. Some prefer to sit and repeat a sound or word over and over. By concentrating on breathing patterns, relaxing, and a focus point, the person meditating can achieve a calm and peaceful mood. Some people find a quiet atmosphere without others to be the best situation. Churches, synagogues, and other places of worship may be preferred by some.

Whether you call it meditation or praying or seeking of the true self, it is a healthy answer to stress. Before conception is the time to learn techniques that will last and benefit you for a lifetime.

Most childbirth classes teach some forms of relaxation and breathing. In essence, they are forms of yoga and meditation. They are used during labor and delivery but perhaps even more, during those difficult times as parents. The lifelong benefits from relaxing through meditation will enhance and enrich coping skills.

## Mental Imagery

We all have the ability to make movies in our minds. We can call up those "films" that actually took place, like a wonderful outing or a beautiful sunset. Relaxation through mental imagery is a wonderful way to unwind. This technique is often used in childbirth classes. The instructor talks the class into taking a trip in their minds, to a peaceful, quiet place.

It is not something that necessarily requires a guide. It can be achieved by oneself. Here is how to proceed:

1. Find a quiet place to sit, lounge, or lie down.

2. If it is comfortable to do so, pull the window shades, and create a nonstimulating atmosphere.

3. Begin with deep cleansing breaths and total relaxation of every body part.

4. Talking to yourself, in your mind, place yourself in a setting of great enjoyment. It may be the beach, the mountains, on a sailboat, or anywhere.

5. With your mind's eye, visualize yourself in that setting. You are alone, content to be so. Continue to take cleansing breaths, and keep your breathing at a slow, steady pace.

6. With each of your senses, experience the setting. Smell the sea breezes, feel the cool spray from the crashing waves, and feel the warm golden sun on every area of your body. The sand under you molds to your body, making a soft bed. Picture yourself nude or dressed but com-

fortable and free. Hear the sea gulls laughing to each other, and the rhythm of the crashing waves. See the long, deserted beach, and feel the enjoyment in the solitude. Taste the salt on your lips, smell the suntan lotion, feel your hair gently blowing across your face and around your neck and shoulders. You feel so relaxed and free.

7. You are feeling the image and have truly removed yourself from your present setting. When you feel the need to return, or leave the beach, then do so. Enjoy it while you are there.

Women in labor are encouraged to learn and master mental imagery skills. During labor, or on any hectic day with your newborn, mental imagery is the coping technique to call on.

### Relax, Relax, Relax

We are told by everyone we meet, "Hey, how about just relaxing?" It sounds so easy, and it is so hard to do. Some people find relaxing possible only with alcohol or drugs. They do not have enough faith in their own relaxation skills.

We are able to relax ourselves without chemicals. Relaxation is essential in yoga, meditation, and mental imagery. Such a simple thing may increase your life expectancy and create a more peaceful existence.

What does it take to truly relax? Try this exercise in controlled relaxation:

1. The first step is to recognize the difference between tension and relaxation.

2. Find a comfortable place. Whether sitting, lying down, or lounging, make sure your feet are off the floor and you are comfortable.

3. Again, begin this exercise with two deep cleansing breaths, in through your nose and out through your mouth.

4. Breathing slowly and regularly, begin by tensing the shoulders. Draw them up to the ears and keep them tense for the count of ten. Then release the tension totally. Feel the difference between the relaxed and tense shoulders. Next do the arms, tensing each separately. Pull each arm up, making a fist, creating complete tension. Release the arms, letting all the tension run out of the fingertips. Repeat this with the legs, buttocks, and even the face.

5. After relaxing each body part, continue the slow, steady breathing. You will be able to recognize the difference between tension and relaxation. You want to feel like a big rag doll sitting or lying wherever you are. No tension, no stress, totally relaxed.

This exercise is especially enjoyable after a long day or if getting to sleep is difficult. In combination with mental imagery, a restful night of sleep is inevitable.

## SELF-ESTEEM AND STRESS

The stress of pregnancy and parenthood can only be made worse if the woman has a poor self-image. Let's face it, how can she handle the criticism, conflict, and constant pressures if she is unable to believe in her capabilities? Women tend to base their self-worth on their performance as employees, as homemakers, mothers, wives, lovers, or daughters.

Self-image plays an important role in emotional health. Good emotional health will allow for coping with stress. Because of the changing role of motherhood, women may experience difficulty in establishing and maintaining self-esteem. Certain principles can be followed to help create a more powerful self-image:

1. Establish a healthy physical state. As discussed previously, good physical health is vital to preconceptional readiness. A healthy body includes good diet and regular exercise. Elimination of chemicals like alcohol, drugs, caffeine, and nicotine are necessary as well. Women who are in good physical condition tend to look better and feel better about themselves.

2. Like yourself. As children growing up, we are encouraged not to think too highly of ourselves. Then, as adolescents, our parents wonder why we do not possess self-confidence. We receive mixed messages. What matters is that as women, we realize we have potential and abilities as well as limitations.

Accept your strengths and capabilities, and learn to believe in yourself. Be realistic in your expectations of yourself and accept your limitations. Do not base your worth on your accomplishments but rather on your very existence. Learn from mistakes; be gentle with yourself, caring, and understanding.

3. Like other people. Liking other people includes accepting them no matter how different they are from you. Acceptance of others creates approval of self. Acceptance is a willingness to at least listen to another point of view, perhaps even learning something new.

4. Establish and maintain a confidant. By having someone to talk to, a relationship is established. Whether it is a friend, lover, spouse, psychotherapist, or a hairdresser, it is an exchange of thoughts and feelings.

Relating is a positive aspect of living. Becoming part of a group is also a healthy activity. In a group setting, people tend to be less occupied with their own problems. Social skills are implemented. Socializing is important for good mental health.

Many pregnant women join prenatal exercise groups for exercise and socialization. Being with other women in the same physical and psychological state is highly therapeutic. Exchanging concerns, fears, and experiences supports the group members in a healthy way.

After the baby is born, new mother groups are available. Some prepared childbirth classes have gone on to start their own support groups in their homes. There is strong evidence telling us that postpartum support is important to head off severe depression.

While 50 to 80 percent of women experience postpartum depression in the first few days after birth, a small percentage continue to experience depression. Strong support by spouse, family, and friends is vital to the new mother.

3. Work and create. Taking satisfaction in a job well done is always therapeutic. Whether working at home or away from home, women desire to do a good job. Feeling positive about work helps boost self-esteem. Once again, it is worth mentioning that self-worth should not be entirely based on work produced, on the job or at home.

Be realistic in your expectations of yourself; do the best you can, and be satisfied. Aldous Huxley once said, "There is only one corner of the universe you can be certain of improving, and that's your own self."

Developing a stronger self-image will strengthen coping skills. Learning to relax and become in tune with your inner self are lifetime skills to be mastered. A strong self will assure you that you can and will be able to handle the stress and challenge of pregnancy and parenthood.

## DYSFUNCTIONAL FAMILIES

As children, we come to our family like blank slates. Our parents, grandparents, siblings, and extended family hold the writing instrument that will create our future. If the knowledge we gain is love, acceptance, hope, and trust, then the future is bright.

Approximately 50 percent of families are considered dysfunctional to some degree. It's like a potter molding a clay vessel. If he works carelessly, cracks form, and the vessel falls apart once heat is applied. People, too, can be like clay vessels, living lives that fall apart under pressure.

Dysfunctional families may include parents who are addicted to alco-

65

hol or drugs. There may be physical or sexual abuse, gambling, overeating, or emotional abandonment. There are even parents who are workaholics. The children of dysfunctional families are never given the chance to work through these painful times, which leads them to become adult "children."

They find their own lives are dysfunctional, either openly or deep inside. Children of alcoholics tend to establish relationships with alcoholics. They tend to possess a low self-worth and may develop a dependent personality.

Millions of people come from dysfunctional families and do not realize who they are. They do not recognize normal. They tend to have tragic relationships, are harsh in self-judgment, and are insecure. They are in pain and influence the world around them. Their pain will affect the next generation, their children.

Looking at the past may be painful for some, but that is how the move ahead begins. Preparing for parenthood includes examining the family from whence we came.

Children raised in dysfunctional homes never really get to know their true selves. They suffer from confusion, chronic unhappiness, difficulty in relating, and guilt. What children need to be healthy includes security, touching, guidance, acceptance, trust, freedom, fun and play, support to grieve, and unconditional love.

Adult children are trying to work through all the tensions of unfinished childhood business. They must deal with their adult conflicts as well. When the two combine, it may cause the person to form compulsions or addictions to alcohol, drugs, food, gambling, sex, abuse, or work. They may suffer from mental illnesses such as depression, personality disorders, psychosis, or criminal behaviors.

While all of this sounds like the end of the road for the adult child, it is just the beginning. On admission and recognition of their past, they can begin to heal and create a more positive life. The multigenerational cycle can be broken and life made brighter for future children.

### Healing the Past for the Future

Healing the dysfunctional past begins by stirring the still waters of our memories. It begins by seeking to discover who the true self is. What starts as pain turns into freedom from the past. Love that has always been there becomes part of the adult child's life.

Turning your back on your dysfunctional family is the first move.

Quite often, the adult child never really leaves home. She is part of the dysfunctional family, unless she breaks away and returns as a functional adult.

This is not always a comfortable thing to do. There is a sense of loss and grieving. Then, there is the realization that you are a survivor of the dysfunctional family. Not only have you survived but you are going to move ahead and make a better life for you, yourself, the people around you, and future generations.

The survivor will feel very much alone at first. That is why therapists and support groups are necessary. While feeling alone, the adult child becomes an adult with insight into who she is. The inner self grows and learns to depend on itself, finding self-worth in spite of the past.

### Finding Help: Who and Why?

Part of the healing process includes learning to open up the Pandora's box of the past. This is not always an easy thing to do alone. Fortunately, therapists and support groups are available. Before signing up for counseling, it is important to do some research.

The telephone is probably the best and most economical place to begin. Most communities have mental health centers that can refer you to mental health resources. Some hotlines are in operation to give immediate support. They are staffed by volunteers.

The community mental health centers are not only economical but have a broad range of professionals involved. A psychiatrist, psychologists, therapists, and social workers make up the staff.

Initially, the person in search of counseling would go for an interview. This serves several purposes. The therapist can assess the client and determine to what degree there is a mental health problem. The client also observes the counselor and decides if she is comfortable with him. This visit does not mean a permanent commitment must be established. It is reasonable to shop around for the right therapist.

It is important to choose a therapist whom you as a woman can feel comfortable talking to. This does not mean you should only see female therapists; there are plenty of male therapists who are sensitive and professional. Asking friends or perhaps a local woman's organization for a list of therapists may help.

The following types of counseling are available.

## Psychiatrists

Psychiatrists are medical doctors who have furthered their education in the area of mental and emotional disturbances. They are qualified to prescribe medications as well as admit patients to hospitals for psychiatric treatment.

They should be board certified or made board eligible by a national examining board. They should be members of the American Psychiatric Association and graduates of a psychotherapy institute. The amount of education they have does not always make them better therapists. Their fees are, on the average, higher than those of other therapists. Some private insurance policies will cover the cost of psychiatric counseling.

## Psychologists

These therapists usually possess master's degrees or doctorates. They are licensed by state boards. They are trained in psychological testing, diagnosis and treatment, psychotherapy, and research. They may have a private practice or work for mental health centers or hospitals. Their fees vary according to their location and the type of practice they are in.

## Psychotherapists

These therapists perform the same work as psychologists and possess the same education. They have not received their state board licensure but are usually preparing for it.

## Social Workers

These graduates of schools of social work are granted master's degrees in social work. They may receive training in either psychiatric, medical, or community social work. They counsel in hospitals, welfare offices, mental health centers, and schools. Their counseling is family oriented. Some states certify social workers to practice independently. It is an asset for a social worker to be a member of the Academy of Certified Social Workers. Their fees are lower than those of other therapists.

## Counselors

Usually found in schools of education, well-trained counselors can be very helpful. And they tend to be more flexible than other types of therapists. They often make referrals as needed and are tuned to a variety of resources.

Most therapists fall under an eclectic heading. They do some analysis but utilize a more directive approach. They tend to give advice, information, and specific instructions. They may also use behavior therapy. They may work with a psychiatrist by accepting referrals after an evaluation.

Choosing a therapist is an important decision. As with any other choice where your valuable time and money are involved, make sure that the one you choose can meet your needs. By deciding to go to a therapist, you are taking another step toward a healthier psychological and emotional life.

### Group Therapy
This form of therapy brings together a group of people with problems in need of exploration. It is conducted by a trained professional. Some positive aspects include a greater amount of support, the opportunity to interact with a variety of people, and receiving good feelings by helping others in the group. One must be comfortable in a group setting, willing to be open and honest with feelings and revealing painful memories or thoughts.

### Support Groups
These groups have formed for support and encouragement of a variety of people with painful lives. Adult Children of Alcoholics, Gamblers Anonymous, Pills Anonymous, Weight Watchers, Alcoholics Anonymous, Al-Anon (for families of alcoholics), Alateen (for teen alcoholics), Parents Anonymous, and Parents Without Partners are just a few support groups that have helped change the lives of countless individuals and families. These groups give hope to participants by demonstrating that others have survived what they are experiencing and are now living fuller lives.

### CHOOSING TO MAKE THE CHANGE
Creating a family involves a true understanding of the creators. We must consider our own mental health as an influencing factor in our children's future. We should not be afraid of our past or feel hopeless.

As adults, we are faced with daily decisions, stress, and ghosts from the past. Everyone wants to succeed and have the best life. We become so involved with careers, jobs, dreams, and relationships that we may be overlooking our true selves.

As potential parents, it is a loving act to learn about ourselves from the inside out. If there is a need for change, do not be afraid to seek help. Stirring up the past may have to be painful in order to create a whole life. Life can be much richer when both physical and mental health are in top form. Alex Carrel said, "Man cannot remake himself without suffering. For he is both the marble and the sculptor."

## SUGGESTED READING

*Unfinished Business*
Maggie Scarf
Ballantine Books, 1980

*Making Peace with Your Parents*
Harold H. Bloomfield, M.D., with Leonard Felder, Ph.D.
Ballantine Books, 1983

*My Mother/My Self*
Nancy Friday
Dell Books, 1987

*The Road Less Traveled*
M. Scott Peck, M.D.
Simon and Schuster, 1978

*In a Different Voice*
Carol Gilligan
Harvard University Press, 1982

*The Troubled People Book*
Paul G. Quinnett
The Continuum Publishing Co., 1982

*Psychology of Women*
Juanita H. Williams
W. W. Norton and Company, Inc., 1977

*Becoming Your Own Parent*
Dennis Wholey
Doubleday, 1988

*Women in Transition*
Andrew DuBrin, Ph.D.
Thomas Publications, 1972

*The Mind-Body Effect*
Herbert Benson, M.D.
Berkeley Publishing Corp., 1979

*The Therapeutic Touch:*
*How to Use Your Hands to Help or to Heal*
Dolores Krieger, Ph.D., R.N.
Prentice-Hall, Inc., 1979

*Responsible Assertive Behavior*
Arthur J. Lange and Patricia Jakubowski
Research Press, Champaign, IL 1976

*Progressive Relaxation*
E. Jacobson
University of Chicago Press, 1938

*Psychotherapy for Women: Treatment Toward Equality*
D. Carter and E. Rawlings, editors
Charles Thomas, 1976

*Stress without Distress*
Hans Celye
New American Library, 1974

*A New Guide to Rational Living*
Albert Ellis and Robert A. Harper
Prentice-Hall, 1975

## RESOURCE GROUPS

Al-Anon Family Groups
1 Park Avenue
New York, NY 10016
212-481-6565

Alateen
1 Park Avenue
New York, NY 10016
212-481-6576

Alcoholics Anonymous
468 Park Avenue South
South New York, NY 10016
212-686-1100

Narcotics Anonymous
P.O. Box 622
Sun Valley, CA 91352
213-764-4880

Parents Without Partners
8807 Colesville Road
Silver Spring, MD 20910
301-588-9354

National Self-Help Resource Center
200 South Street N.W.
Washington, D.C. 20009
202-388-5704

National Self-Help Clearinghouse
33 W. 42nd Street
New York, NY 10036
212-840-7606

Mental Health Assocition
National Headquarters
1800 North Kent Street
Arlington, VA 22209
703-528-6405

American Association of Marriage and Family Counselors
225 Yale Avenue
Claremont, CA 91711
714-621-4749

Family Resource Coalition
230 North Michigan Avenue
Suite 1625
Chicago, IL 60601
312-726-4750

Family Service America
1170 West Lake Park Drive
Milwaukee, WI 53224
414-359-2111

Women's Health Communications
4512 Springfield Avenue
Philadelphia, PA 19143
No telephone listing available.

National Council of Community Mental Health Centers
6101 Montrose Road, Suite 360
Rockeville, MD 20852
301-984-6200

American Institute of Stress
124 Park Avenue
Yonkers, NY 10703
914-963-1200

CHAPTER 6

# MEN AND FATHERHOOD

*"There are no absolutes in raising children. In any stressful*
*situation, fathering is always a roll of the dice. The game may be*
*messy, but I have never found one with more rewards and joys."*

—Bill Cosby

## FATHERHOOD

Just as women realize that pregnancy and parenthood bring major life
changes, fathers know they too will never be the same. Fatherhood
means different things to different men. Culturally, it has meant that the
father is the provider of food and shelter. He is the one who is expected
to be strong and financially responsible for his family. These established
standards do not always support a man's desire to be involved in his partner's pregnancy or in an equal parenting experience.

What is his reaction to the prospect of becoming a father? If he
demonstrates an interest or even enthusiasm, you may be getting somewhere. Becoming a father begins with how willing he is to take this first
step into parenthood. Talk about feelings and perceptions of fatherhood.

What role does he see himself playing once conception has been
accomplished? Does he plan to accompany you to your prenatal
checkups and childbirth classes? Most important, does he plan to be at
the birth, or does he think that is carrying this thing just too far? His
generation generally did not have for a role model a father who attended
the birth of his children.

Fathers at one time were exiled to the waiting room of the hospital to
smoke cigarettes, drink coffee, and pace the floor. Oh, yes, and act nervous. That is the Hollywood rendition of what having a baby was like for
the father. Still, men of the 1980s are not quite sure of their role in this
whole event and need their partners' understanding and some education.

### Prerecorded Messages

For men, there seems to be a fairly rigid set of rules that determines
their outcome as adult men. It all goes back to how much of a human

being the little boy was allowed to be versus the little man he was
expected to be.

"Boys don't play with dolls," "Don't cry when you fall down; get up,
little man," "You're not hurt," and "Don't be such a sissy," are just part
of the collection of messages boys receive from society. Boys are not
encouraged to be sensitive, vulnerable, tender, or to need anyone else. It
may take some effort and even painful moments for a man to work
through those prerecorded messages of his past. A loving and understanding partner can make the transition more bearable.

Change does not occur overnight and should not be expected of the
man who is chosen to be your child's father. It is just not practical to
divorce or leave someone because they lack the characteristics you
desire in a father-to-be. Communication is necessary from the
beginning.

### Role Models

While role models do play an important part in our lives, they do not
have to have the last say in our success as men and women or as parents.
A man may feel the need to develop stronger self-esteem if he comes
from a dysfunctional family (see chap. 5). It is important for him to feel
like an equal partner in this life-changing decision. Listen to his concerns from the very beginning and reassure him. Keeping the lines of
communication open is very important for his development as a father
and your development as parents.

Demonstrating your support in his search for understanding of
fatherhood is vital. When you become pregnant, you will want the same
kind of understanding and support. In fact, studies indicate that a
woman who receives support from the father of the baby both psychologically and emotionally develops a greater sense of competency in her
ability to mother. So it can be beneficial to you both to communicate,
understand, support, and believe in each other. It is a healthy foundation
for building your home.

### What Shape Is He In?

He said yes. He thinks it would be great to have a baby. So, is he ready
physically? Sure, he is not the one who will be pregnant, but his health
is still an important factor.

Researchers have proven that the man's health has a definite
influence on conception. Such factors as alcohol, cigarettes, and infec-

tions have been documented as determinants in the success of healthy reproduction.

The chemical structure of alcohol, for example, can influence the quality of sperm. It not only changes the sperm but causes infertility in some practicing alcoholics. The alcohol affects the prostate gland and irritates it. This irritation produces extra mucous, which does not allow the sperm to be mobile. If they cannot move freely and seek out the egg, then fertilization cannot occur. Alcohol also affects the shape and formation of the sperm. Normal, healthy sperm have a challenge getting to the egg. What chances do malformed sperm have in this highly competitive mission? Not much.

Smoking is another indulgence that men should consider stopping before they attempt to take part in conception. Some researchers believe sperm quality is affected by nicotine. While they may debate this issue, it cannot be denied that a healthier body is one without nicotine.

What about the prospective father's general physical health? Is he overweight, out of shape, a nutritional disaster area? Well, no need to lament. The idea of working together on this preconceptional plan is to encourage one another.

We as a society have been bombarded with health information. TV shows portray fit and virile men as the main characters. Just as women feel they must live up to these Hollywood standards, so do men. Becoming Mr. Universe does not necessarily have to be his goal. Rather, like you, he should look at his present health and decide on a plan of action to become a healthier father-to-be.

Having a mate who is willing to undergo improvement on behalf of the baby-to-be is a step in the right direction. Improved nutrition complete with vitamins will help improve his health and even his sperm. Men who suffer from agglutination, or clumping, of sperm, preventing the sperm from reaching the egg, can add Vitamin C to their diet to treat this disorder. Vitamin E has also been known to help increase fertility. If there is a fertility problem, it is best to seek medical help. (See chap. 13.)

Men should assess their workplace for potential exposure to any radiation or chemical influences. Some men who served in the military in Vietnam were exposed to the defoliant Agent Orange. There have been debates on the effect this exposure may have had on the reproductive abilities of these soldiers. Exposing the reproductive tract directly, as with alcohol, smoking, and drugs, or indirectly, as with radiation and chemicals, can influence sperm quality and fertility, perhaps even more than is realized.

## FATHERHOOD ONE MORE TIME

What if this is his second family? Let us say he married young, had three kids, and divorced. He fell in love with you, and you married him. Although he is ten years your senior, you decide you long to have children of your own. What influences will this situation have on your maternal hopes and dreams? Will he become the expert in all areas of your pregnancy, delivery, and child care, or will he fail to show an interest at all? He has done this before, so what's the big deal?

The thrill of pregnancy and the anticipation of labor and delivery should be granted to any woman who wants it. If her mate has had the experience, he should be encouraged to give helpful advice in a loving manner. If your partner has a tendency to compare you with his ex-wife, beware. Talk it over with him, explaining that you are willing to accept helpful, factual information to make your pregnancy the best it can be.

A positive point about a man with an established family is that you can observe his parenting skills. Does he nurture his kids, or is he a drill sergeant? Before conception is the time to discuss how you as a couple will parent your child. It is important that he realize that your child will be different from his other offspring. That is a vital aspect for him to consider and accept. Discuss with him how you plan to raise your child. Review some of your conflicting beliefs with him.

Discussions like this are not meant to be challenges to his paternal role. They are golden opportunities to help direct you both into better parenting. He has the experience, and you both have a chance to begin a new parenting adventure together.

## WHAT ABOUT WORK?

From one generation to the next, fathers have graduated from being excluded from the delivery to assisting the doctor and cutting the umbilical cord. An estimated 80 to 90 percent of American fathers are now in attendance at the birth of their children. This kind of initial involvement tends to draw the family together. The man learns to appreciate firsthand what his mate undergoes as she is transformed into a mother through the birth process.

Circumstances do arise which prevent couples from sharing the birth experience. The experts on bonding may even try to make the absent father feel like a failure for not witnessing the birth of his child. Psychologists are saying that there is no evidence to support such radical views. Fathers who do not attend, by choice or due to uncontrollable circumstances, can be as close to their child as those who do attend.

Ellen became pregnant while Matt was a third-year medical resident. Matt recalls phoning Ellen while she was in labor in one hospital and he was on duty in another hospital across town. They understood that this was what Matt's job involved. Being apart for perhaps days at a time was part of their life-style, and they had to work around it. Ellen delivered their son and was waiting for Matt to arrive when he was off duty.

Because not everyone has a 9 to 5 husband or partner, women learn to adjust their lives. Adjusting includes accepting their schedules and working with it. Before conception, discuss how his work and starting a family may conflict. If you find too many conflicts, maybe conception should be delayed. If he is still in college or interested in climbing a few more rungs on the career ladder, consider postponing pregnancy until a better time in your lives.

Some women with workaholic husbands may view having a baby as an answer to loneliness. But instead they may experience resentment toward the mate and the child. A partner with a demanding, time-consuming job is not able to parent on a totally equal basis. It results in the mother sometimes feeling like a single parent.

What are the choices when his job demands more of him than you want to give? Here are a few possibilities.

## Alternate Plan

What are other areas of work that could pay the same and give him more regular hours? Would he need to return to school for further education? After the baby arrives, would it make more sense for you to return to work and for him to remain home with the baby? If your job pays well and has regular hours, perhaps it is a reasonable consideration.

## Benefits

Some jobs are worth tolerating just for the benefits. Many couples are checking out benefits even before pay scales when taking jobs. It is difficult to pass up a job that has complete medical and dental coverage, four weeks paid vacation, paid holidays, and ten sick days. It may mean a compromise in time for good benefits.

Careers are important for financial security. Whatever arrangements you and your partner can make to allow for more time together should be made. Men should be aware of their paternity rights at their place of employment. Some places will allow them a leave of absence after the baby is born. The adjustments of parenthood can be difficult at times, and the support you find from each other is important.

## GETTING HIM INVOLVED

If he agrees to take part in conception, must he participate any further? This may be the unspoken attitude of some men. They may feel that because the woman is the one who is pregnant, there is nothing more they can do. After all, how often is the expectant father fussed over in social or family settings? He needs to be reassured that he is an equal partner in the pregnancy, childbirth, and parenthood experience.

It is not uncommon to have fathers bring reading material to child birth classes anticipating boredom. They are not sure why they are there or how their wives convinced them to attend. Both mothers and fathers are surprised to learn just how vital dad is in the process of labor, delivery, and parenting.

Men who choose not to attend classes or the birth of the child may have fears they are unable to share. Seeing the woman they love in pain is not always an easy sight. Many men think that the blood may cause them to become weak, even faint. It is for these reasons that education is so important. Once they have an understanding of labor and delivery, they are able to become effective support persons. In fact, many fathers admit being so involved with the mother, helping her with breathing techniques and relaxation, that they are not at all bothered.

Men who are excluded from the birth of their child by circumstance have a more difficult time. In an emergency cesarean section, time is of the essence, and the health team may not have time to supervise the father. The man who must experience this type of emergency situation tends to feel out of control. He may feel terrified for his wife and their child and not receive the necessary support. This is not particularly the best way to begin fatherhood.

What is your partner's job description as Daddy? Does he do baby baths? Does he do bottles? Does he do diapers? What exactly does he plan to do? It is a good idea to find out how he perceives his role in this parental partnership. It is not necessary or wise to bully him into parenting. If he is encouraged and praised, he will probably be more willing to participate. He may even find it enjoyable to care for his baby.

As mothers, we know that fathers can meet all the needs of a new baby, except for breast-feeding. In fact, studies show that babies do actively become attached to their fathers. Attachment involves promoting contact between father and baby. That makes sense. In fact, the more involved the father is in the pregnancy, birth, and day-to-day care, the more tolerant he is toward the child in general.

Becoming a father requires on-the-job training. It takes time and requires patience and loving support from his partner. Any sound relationship requires getting to know each other and learning to accept one another. For father and child, the same advice applies.

## TALKING THROUGH FEELINGS

It is not only women who worry about their pregnancy, what labor and delivery will be like, and their ability to mother. Men have great concerns for their partners' welfare, and they worry about their capabilities as fathers.

It makes sense for the couple to communicate freely. By talking through the fears, concerns, and anxieties, both may find reassurance and comfort. Areas that may be of concern and should be discussed preconceptionally are as follows.

1. Age: Does he feel he is too old, too young, or just right?

2. Job: Is his job time consuming? Does it take him away from home frequently? Does he bring his work home with him? Are you required to contribute to his career, through dinners, cocktail parties, or otherwise entertaining VIPs? If so, how does a baby fit into this setting?

3. Income and Benefits: Will his job support the family? If you do not return to work, by choice or necessity, will his job pay the bills and provide good benefits? Is he able to take vacation time when he wants, or does he have to request time off in advance? Babies come when they are ready. Is he eligible for parental leave, similar to maternity leave?

4. Role Change: How will he feel about changing from husband/lover to father? Will it be a confining role for him? Is he willing to be an equal parent? Is he concerned with being a "good" dad, and if so, what does that mean to him?

5. Sexuality: Will parenting make a difference in his feelings about sex with you? Does he think privacy will be affected by the birth of a child? Does he understand that some women have a decreased interest in sex after the birth? Would he be willing to be patient and sensitive to your needs at this time?

6. Baby Concerns: Does he worry about the baby's health? Is he concerned about birth defects, a complicated labor and delivery, or even your death or the baby's?

7. Philosophies: How does he feel about his wife breast-feeding in public? What are his thoughts on discipline, education, spiritual upbringing? Does it matter if it is a boy or a girl? If so, why? What are his concerns about bringing a child into the world? What are some of his dreams for his child?

8. Increased Responsibilities: Does the idea of a long-term commitment to his child bother him? Is he willing to take time if the baby is ill and needs to be seen by the doctor? What if you are sick? Will he be home to help, or are you on your own?

9. The Birth Process: Is he interested in attending childbirth classes and learning what this is all about? Does he feel forced to attend, or does he feel out of place? After all, his mom did it alone, shouldn't you be able to? Does he think he will faint or get sick during the delivery? What is it about the birth that might bother him the most?

10. Health and Longevity: Is he concerned about any health problems? If he has a disability, does he fear it will inhibit his paternal capabilities? Is he concerned with any family history of birth defects? Is there a history of a genetic disease in his family? Does he worry about his own fertility, fearing that he may not even be able to father a child?

## WHAT A DIFFERENCE A DAD MAKES

A man can either father a child or be a father to a child. The difference is obvious. Fatherhood, like motherhood, can be quite frightening the first time. Men may find it difficult to express their anxieties. As their partners and friends, we must encourage them to do so and accept what they say.

Before conception is the time to help him work through his concerns. Together, you can seek out information that may ease some of the fears. The most important step in creating a baby is to create a mother and father who are truly prepared.

## SUGGESTED READING

*Father's Influence on Children*
Marshall L. Hamilton
Nelson-Hall, 1977

*The Male Machine*
Marc Fergen Fastean
Delta Books, 1975

*Why Can't Men Open Up?*
Steven Naifeh and Gregory White Smith
Clarkson N. Potter, Inc., Publishers, 1984

*Men and Marriage*
Elizabeth C. Mooney
Franklin Watts, Inc., 1985

*Who Will Raise the Children? New Options for Fathers (and Mothers)*
James A. Levine
J. B. Lippincott Company, 1976

*Expectant Fathers*
Sam Bittman and Sue Rosenberg Zalk, Ph.D.
Ballantine Books, 1978

*Fatherhood*
Bill Cosby
Berkley Books, 1986

## RESOURCE GROUPS

Family Service Association of America
44 East 23rd Street
New York, NY 10010
212-674-6100

Single Dad's Hotline
P.O. Box 4842
Scottsdale, AZ 85258
602-998-0980

# CHAPTER 7

# FROM THE GROUND UP
## The Family Foundation

*"The family you come from isn't as important as the family you're going to have."*

—Ring Lardner

## IF BABY COULD CHOOSE, WOULD HE CHOOSE YOU?

We know that babies have no choice in who their parents will be. But what if they did? Would you and your partner be chosen? If you do believe you are qualified, will you be able to provide a secure family foundation?

In previous chapters, the importance of examining your own life and making changes was stressed. Men and women need to possess self-confidence as individuals in order to create a strong couple. You and your partner should strive to support each other and treat each other with respect and dignity.

Children draw strength and find security in a home where the parents have solid footing. Children also base their treatment of people on what they see at home. For example, a son will benefit from seeing his father respect and honor his mother. The same goes for a girl seeing her mother working with her father on decisions and projects.

Every woman planning for a baby worries about being a good parent. What are good parents? Do they ever get angry, frustrated, or resentful? They sure do. Often we set our expectations too high. Then, when we cannot possibly meet them, we feel we have failed. Parents-to-be must set realistic expectations for themselves. Here I will discuss ways in which you can build a solid family foundation.

## MARRIAGE: YES OR NO?

While it is necessary for two people to create a child, it is not necessary for a married couple to raise a child. At one time, according to social standards, it was all but required to be married before the baby arrived. Patterns in marriage and social expectations are changing.

Couples are living together unmarried and, if they marry, are doing so later in life. According to 1984 statistics, the average marriage age for women is 22.8 years old and for men is 24.6 years old. Both are waiting to finish their education before making the legal commitment.

Many couples continue to live together quite happily for years. These couples may find the bonds of matrimony just a little too confining but enjoy an exclusive relationship.

So which is better? The couple must decide. But when it comes to going one step further, to having a baby, there are more factors to consider. The following lists may help you start thinking about this choice.

## Marriage
### Advantages
- Commitment should keep the relationship exclusive.
- Society prefers marriage before children.
- Marriage gives the child legal security.
- It is easy to walk away from conflicts. Couples are more likely to work through problems.
- When there is illness, commitment is more supportive.
- Worry-free sex is more likely in a monogamous relationship.
- Financial security is provided within marriage.
- Love is developed, changes, and with time, matures.

### Disadvantages
- Restricts other relationships.
- The husband may feel the need to dominate in a traditional sense.
- If there are two careers, the woman may have to sacrifice hers before he will his.
- One partner may be less responsible with money than the other.
- Women may be stuck with household duties if an equitable system is not established.
- One partner may outgrow the other over time.
- Partners can easily take each other for granted.
- Romance and sex may get stale.

## Living Together
### Advantages
- There is no need to commit to each other legally.
- If careers go opposite ways, there is no need to sacrifice career for marriage.

- Living together provides time to get to know each other before a commitment takes place.
- The couple can develop their relationship because they want to, not out of legal obligation.
- They can easily remain individuals in name, finances, assets, and so forth.

## Disadvantages
- There is less legal protection for mother and child if the relationship breaks up.
- The relationship may be too easily dissolved if careers conflict.
- It is too easy to look for flaws and problems and consider separating.
- It may be difficult to define the relationship to yourselves and others.
- If one wants to marry eventually and the other does not, conflict develops.
- If one or the other is not convinced of the commitment, he or she may feel a need for more private time.

There are legal considerations also. It is important to make a choice based on the welfare of the child. While a woman may not need marriage for security, what about a child? If you are not married and the relationship dissolves, then the baby may become your responsibility.

Let us say that things get messy and you need child support money. What legal recourse do you have if there is no legal bond between you and your partner? Maybe his name is on the birth certificate, but is that enough to receive support? Child support laws vary from state to state, and this should be checked carefully before considering a child outside of marriage.

Whatever arrangements you make—to live together, to marry, or to live apart and raise the child together—the choice should be given serious thought and made together. There are three people involved, and one has no say in the matter. The child is in need of your well-thought-out decision that will ultimately affect him or her for a lifetime.

It may be difficult to think about a baby-yet-to-be and make decisions for him. That is what preconceptional planning is all about. It means trying to project into the future and anticipate what you think are the important issues that will mold the future for your child.

## YOU DIAPER, I'LL WATCH

"Hazel, the baby smells funny," Harry called from the living room. He had volunteered to rock baby Tommy to sleep after Hazel fed him. The big game was on TV, he had his favorite beer at his side, and now a baby with an odor.

"Okay, Harry, I'll be right there. I'm cooking your favorite, baked lasagna with stuffed grape leaves," Hazel responded.

"Ah, come on Hazel, the game's getting ready to start, and this smell is awful. The whole room is beginning to reek. My beer is going to taste funny now. Please hurry," Harry whined.

"I'll be in as soon as I get the freshly baked bread out of the oven, dear. I'm sorry honey," Hazel apologized as she came running into the living room and scooped little Tommy out of Harry's arms.

"Gee, Hazel, I really don't mind helping out with Tommy, but come when I call for you, OK? Hey, when you're done with him, get me another beer."

"Yes dear," Hazel said as she and the baby left the room.

What is wrong with this family scene? If we could step into this scenario, what would we say to Hazel? How about, "Get real, Hazel, tell that husband of yours to get up and change that baby himself."

What would you say to Harry? "Do you want to eat your meal or wear it, Harry?" This may just be the opening line to many more if Harry were the typical father of the 1980s.

This extreme illustration is not as common nowadays but may still be lived out in some homes. If this type of inequality is taking place, then there is a lack of cooperative parenting in the family foundation.

Two things happen if there is not equal parenting. The woman feels overloaded and develops resentment for both father and baby. And, if allowed, the father can feel left out and unimportant. He, too, can develop resentments toward the baby. So in order for baby to receive a fair deal, parents should discuss care giving before conception.

Sharing the household and child care duties is healthier than assigning them. The advantage of sharing is that each person fills in wherever the need is. If a dad like Harry does not do diapers, then everybody is upset if the baby messes and mom is unavailable. Both parents can learn from the very beginning to diaper, bathe, feed, dress, burp, and calm a fussy baby. Learning together makes parenting an equal endeavor. Besides, two adults can certainly figure out how the car seat works, can't they?

The only task that is truly exclusive to the mother is breast-feeding. This does not mean that dad is off the hook at mealtime. If baby begins to cry, dad can change him and take him to mom. He can help her get comfortable and perhaps bring her a glass of juice or milk to drink while she nurses. This arrangement works well for night feedings as well. Mom can stay in bed and rest, while dad prepares baby and brings him to mom. Something so simple means much to the mother of a baby who is nursing every two or three hours.

Learning to parent together does not mean you are clones. You and your partner will probably have your own ways of performing the same task. Diapering has certain steps to it, but everyone does it just a little differently. Doing it differently does not mean it is done wrong.

Carol and Bill knew nothing about caring for a newborn. Neither had any experience prior to the birth of their daughter, Trudy. They did know that sharing the child care was important to them. Their techniques in caring for Trudy were different and yet equally effective.

Carol liked to rock Trudy when giving her the bottle. About every five minutes, Carol would stop and burp her. She would place the infant over her shoulder and gently pat her back until she burped. She would then feed Trudy some more milk. This technique worked well for Trudy and Carol. Bill preferred feeding Trudy for longer periods of time. He would then walk with Trudy and jiggle her up and down as he sang her songs or talked softly to her. This was what worked for Bill and Trudy.

If the same basic task is performed, what difference does style make? It is good for you and your partner to discuss understanding each other's choice in techniques. If the baby is being cared for safely and efficiently, and he offers no complaints, then relax. It is a common symptom of new parents to be anxious about doing things "just right." Do what works for you as individuals, as a couple, and as a family.

## THE BUILDING BLOCKS FOR A STRONG FOUNDATION

Sharing parenthood involves areas like discipline, spiritual upbringing, philosophies, child care arrangements, and hopes for the future. It may seem early to consider which college the baby-yet-to-be will attend. But if you and your partner have extremely different opinions even now, what will change them? Below are some of the areas to be considered before the child is born.

## Discipline

This is probably the most difficult task undertaken by parents. Whether the parents believe in spanking or not, a child needs some type of guidance. What type of discipline was practiced in your homes? Did both parents correct the child, or was one the primary disciplinarian? In some homes, the father is designated to perform all the discipline. Even if the offense took place at noon, discipline was not meted out until dad got home from work. For others, whenever the offense occurred, the nearest parental hand did the deed.

Of course, you and your partner may not always agree on the severity of the punishment. When children get older, they delight in seeing mom and dad go at it because they cannot agree on which punishment should follow breaking the neighbor's window. Can't you just see a child's face as he watches his parents argue over what to do with him? Maybe his folks will forget about it once they are on speaking terms again. So much for sticking together and mutual agreement.

Some people just naturally believe in chastising a child for wrongdoings, because "that's the way we were raised." That tradition-based attitude needs to be discussed. If one parent believes in physical punishment and the other does not, then there needs to be serious negotiation. When parents do not agree on guidelines for their child, there can be a disintegration of the family foundation.

Developing discipline is a slow, gradual process. Newborns, of course, can do no wrong, nor do they wish to. As a child grows and understands her true power as a little person, she begins to explore and test. This is when parents need to be in agreement on guidelines. What is extremely helpful is to understand the mind of a child (see chap. 9).

So often, in our own frustration as parents, we view a child's actions as deliberate and spiteful, which are adult traits. "She did that on purpose. That little brat broke my ceramic horse because she is angry. She has a temper that needs to be curbed."

Is it possible for a one-year-old to reason through a situation and evaluate the reaction to her action?

"Hmmm, nice ceramic horse you have here, Mom. I understand you and Dad purchased this on your honeymoon in Canada. It really is quite lovely, all black and shiny. It holds a particular interest to me because of its sparkling emerald green eyes. It is light enough for me to pick up, and yet heavy enough to make a wonderful sound as I pound it on your glass top coffee table. Listen to this, Mom (Bang, bang, CRASH). Whoops."

The mind of a child says if it feels good, do it, if it sounds good, make the noise, and if it tastes good, eat it. Why not?

You and your partner should be prepared to discipline your children. Discuss your feelings, experiences, and concerns about the correction of children. There is an ample supply of books by leading experts in child care. Whatever is decided, implement your choice as a team.

## Spiritual Upbringing

Here is an area of your life that can arouse disagreement. It is a sensitive and intense subject that is based on personal beliefs and convictions. At this point in your relationship, spirituality probably has been discussed. You are probably aware of your partner's beliefs. If not, now is the time to talk about it.

Most families have some type of spiritual orientation. How important is spiritual life to you as an individual, as a couple, and as parents-to-be? Do you follow traditional family beliefs by choice or because of pressure from parents? Have you ever considered following another path?

Instilling some type of spiritual background into your children seems important to the average couple. Because our country is based on religious freedom, there are any number of religions to choose from. Some ethnic groups possess strong ties to certain religions. Some families have such strong ties to one church that it seems almost forbidden to try something else. As a couple who may desire to break away, you and your partner have the right and freedom to do so. Some couples may seek a church or religion that neither belongs to. Some couples may choose to follow a spiritual path that is nontraditional or none at all.

This is an area of life worth examining. And at times, your children will ask many profound questions. What happens to you after you die? What happened to our pet dog after he died? Who made the Earth, sun, and stars? What is this big, wide world all about, and how did I get here? Preparation for such questions can be made by discussing your beliefs with each other.

## Philosophies and Values

Everyone has a theory or view of the way the world is in general or in a personal sense. Most couples are aware of each other's views and either accept or reject them. Fortunately, we are allowed to have our own personal philosophies, but they can become an issue when a child is involved. Parents tend to force their views on their offspring, intentionally or otherwise.

You and your partner, as potential parents, must dig deep inside to recognize what areas will affect your kids. The topic of freedom for children is one potential area of conflict. How much freedom is too much? Should children be allowed to explore and learn freely? Do they need our guidance and input on a constant basis? Is it our duty to impart our values to them or to teach them both sides of every issue?

Here are a few healthy guidelines to use in teaching values to your children:

1. Expose a child to as much as possible—cultural, social, political, natural, and spiritual.

2. Recognize your own convictions on different issues.

3. Let your children be different from you. Present both sides of every issue, and allow them to reason through their choices.

4. Understand that convictions are related to the time. The youth of the 1960s were harassed because they were different from their parents. Your children will have unique issues to confront as they grow up. Refrain from using the classic line, "When I was a kid, we did thus and such."

5. Do not try to live out personal fantasies through your child. While sports are a wonderful device to keep kids busy, it is not fair to push your child into them just because you were a star quarterback.

6. When it comes to education and careers, support and guide them in their choice.

7. Be aware of a natural tendency toward being sexist in your child's career choice. Why not encourage your daughter to be a doctor instead of a nurse? Why not encourage your son to become an artist or writer, as opposed to a top executive?

8. Accept your child for who she is each day of her life. It is easy to get caught up in what she should be or could be, rather than just who she is, just the way she is.

## Hopes and Dreams and Superkids

With the birth of a baby, parents become infatuated with their child's accomplishments. Baby books are kept like sacred journals. Each first is recorded, each tooth is documented, and each holiday card from the grandparents carefully secured to the pages.

It is a wonder to behold when this helpless little being rolls over, sits up, and takes that first step. These are milestones for both parent and child. What would it be like if parents, blessed with a healthy baby, were just not satisfied?

"Jerry, I read in a magazine that babies that sit up at three months are more likely to do better on their college SATs than babies who sit up at four months," new mother Kate said.

"Is that right? I heard from my colleagues that if you read the dictionary to your baby while you are pregnant, it will talk sooner than other kids," Jerry noted.

"Public TV had a show on the other day about the effect of apple juice on a child's musical capability," Kate said.

"Is that right, Kate? Hmmm, where is Jeffrey's bottle? I'll get the apple juice."

While it is natural to want the best for our offspring, things should be kept in perspective. Competition within our society is strong. Parents can get caught in that trap if not careful. By believing that they are helping their children by pushing them at an early age, parents are deceiving themselves and harming their children.

Parenthood is a job that everyone wants to do well. Keeping a perspective of what that means is vital. Pushing a child, causing stress in his life, and setting him up for frustration is not healthy parenting.

Parents vary, possessing individual values and backgrounds. Education, life-style, and success levels determine what pressures will be placed on their children. Parents-to-be must be aware of the likelihood that they will expect great things from their child. It is important to keep in mind that each child is different and talented in his own unique way. Your child will differ from other kids of the same age, gender, and family and will be different from you.

## STRONG FOUNDATIONS BUILD HAPPY KIDS

Families are responsible for turning a baby into a socially acceptable human being. Sounds easy, doesn't it? Throughout a person's life, security and acceptance most often are sought from his own family. The first five or six years of a child's life are spent being transformed. The stage is set for the child, adolescent, and young adult's lifetime.

The realization of such a powerful family influence on kids can be frightening. Establishing a strong family foundation should be attempted before conception. How can that be done before there are children? Simple. Think of yourselves as a family just waiting to happen. Consider the adjustments to be made in moving from a couple to a family. Observe families and how they function today versus other generations. Realize that times do change and that what was good for us as kids may not work for our children.

There are no easy answers for helping our children with the pressures they will encounter in this world. One thing remains true: the family foundation, like any structure expected to last for years and years, needs to be solid. A family with its feet planted firmly on the ground will be the haven a child will always seek out for love, acceptance, and a sense of security.

Statistics show that 50 percent of all first-time marriages will end in divorce. This means that half of all families will eventually dissolve. If not done sensitively and smoothly, children suffer and may have long-term emotional problems.

The choice to create a family is serious, indeed. If you and your partner know preconceptionally that yours is an unstable relationship, seek help in the form of counseling. It is a kind, loving act for preparing for parenthood.


## SUGGESTED READING

*Becoming Parents*
Sandra Sohn Jaffe and Jack Viertel
Antheneum, 1979

*On Becoming a Family*
T. Berry Brazelton, M.D.
Dell, 1982

*Traits of a Healthy Family*
Dolores Curran
Ballantine Books, 1983

*Living with Your New Baby*
Elly Rakowitz and Gloria S. Rubin
Berkley Books, 1978

*Hide or Seek*
Dr. James Dobson
Fleming H. Revell Co., 1974

*Women, Wives, Mothers: Values and Options*
J. Bernard
Aldine Publishing, 1975

*Dual Career Families*
Robert Rapoport, and Rhona Rapoport
Penguin Books, 1971

## RESOURCE GROUPS

Coping with the Overall Pregnancy/Parenting Experience (COPE)
37 Clarendon Street
Boston, MA 02116
617-357-5588

Family Development Program
Children's Hospital
Boston, MA 02146
617-734-6000, ext. 3275

American Institute for Family Relations
4942 Vineland Avenue N.
Hollywood, CA
No telephone listing available.

# CHAPTER 8

# SINGLE PARENTING
## Mom and Dad in One

*"Children are a great comfort in your old age—
and they help you reach it faster, too."*
—Lionel Kauffman

## AN UNEXPECTED PREGNANCY

Terry could not have been happier. She was pregnant with Dave's child. Although he was not finished with his tour of duty in Thailand, that was all right with Terry. She and Dave had planned to marry in two months. They would be a family and would all live happily ever after.

Not long after discovering that she was pregnant, Terry received a letter from Dave. He had been thinking about their relationship and was not sure they should marry. In fact, he thought they should see other people before making such a serious commitment as marriage. Dave took the letter one step further and told Terry that he was seeing someone else. Of course, he still cared for Terry and wished her the best of luck. But luck was not exactly what she needed at this time in her life.

Women from all walks of life may find themselves pregnant at what seems like the wrong time of their lives. This is nothing new for women. The refining of birth control and choosing to abstain from intercourse have helped decrease the number of unwanted pregnancies. And yet, they still occur.

The unfortunate reality is that after a sexual encounter, a man can walk away and possibly deny it ever took place. The woman, in doubt, waits for a period that never comes. She lives in fear of the day when her body begins the changes that come with the child that grows within her. What might otherwise be a joyful beginning of new life turns into a living nightmare for the woman. She is faced with decisions that will change her life and that of her child forever.

Another woman may view an unplanned pregnancy as a challenge. Perhaps if her life is stable and her career established, if she has a strong support system and is financially sound, the child would be a welcome addition to her life. Neither situation is ideal, but neither is impossible to handle.

Decisions are not always easy to make when you know it is for two of you. Pregnancy is a difficult time to make choices. Hormonal changes themselves create emotional changes. It is physiological and frustrating. For some, especially for younger and lower-income women, like Terry, there would seem to be limited choices.

Abortion is a choice that was legalized in the 1974 Supreme Court decision, *Roe vs. Wade*. It has been a source of controversy between members of pro-choice and pro-life groups ever since. Whether it is good or bad, moral or unjust, it is an available choice to eliminate an unwanted pregnancy. In summer 1989, the Supreme Court ruled to allow each state to establish its own laws governing abortion. Once again the issue of how much control a woman has over her own body is resurrected. It is important for the woman considering abortion to learn the laws in her state of residence concerning her right to an abortion.

Women choosing abortion have made their decision based on their personal situations. Motherhood at sixteen is traumatic for even the best supported young woman. The psychological pressures and physical stress of pregnancy can change a young woman's life forever. Undergoing an abortion could be an equally life-changing experience.

Either choice, to have an abortion or to give birth to the child, is difficult. The woman must consider all her options, seek counseling, and make the choice that is right for her.

If a woman decides to give birth to the child, what about adoption? This is another difficult choice for a pregnant woman to make. It involves going through an entire pregnancy, labor, and birth. It also includes giving up legal rights to the child she bore. While advocates of adoption view this as a loving act to be made for the child, it does not take away the pain of permanent separation of mother and child. It does allow the child to have a more solid foundation on which it can grow, and perhaps even a better life.

## BEING A SINGLE PARENT

For some women, pregnancy is a desired state. They realize that while they may not be ready to get married, or even commit to a relationship with a man, they would like to be mothers.

Single mothers are not unusual. In 1986, single parent households made up 8.9 million of the families in our nation. Most of these single parent households are the result of the increased divorce rate. Others are a result of women choosing to raise children by themselves. In some cases, women have chosen to exclude the child's father from their lives. In 1986, 30 percent of the single mother households were women who never married. Let's examine some of the advantages and disadvantages of single parenting.

## Advantages:

1. Mothers may have more time for their children since they do not have to be wives as well. In a bad relationship, it is difficult to switch successfully from unhappy wife to happy mother.

2. Development of a special, perhaps closer mother-child relationship can occur. Mother and child learn to help and give to one another. Mothers are able to find joy in their children in the midst of turmoil. The child's natural innocence and goodness help mothers cope.

3. There is no partner to disagree with over child rearing. One person makes the rules and regulations. There is generally less conflict in the household. Mothers find a positive change in their relationships with their children.

4. Mothers who are leaving a situation in which the father has been immature or tyrannical may find child rearing alone less stressful, and the children will benefit from this more positive atmosphere.

5. Learning to be independent benefits the woman, making her a stronger role model for her children. Children learn to appreciate self-sufficiency in this situation.

## Disadvantages:

1. It can be difficult to keep house, work outside the home, and give kids time. It may be necessary to sacrifice a clean house for time with the children.

2. It is almost vital to have a network of friends or family to rely on for emotional and maybe even financial support.

3. It may be difficult to find peace and quiet for self in a home where you are the total care giver.

4. Dating and sexuality may be compromised by maternal responsibility.

5. Pursuit of support from the child's father may be a never-ending struggle. Be prepared.

6. It may not always be easy to understand how children perceive the situation.

7. Dreams of that house in the country, further education, or having a significant other may be postponed. Making ends meet is the focus.

A woman who decides to raise her child outside marriage must seriously consider if she wants the father in the picture. Some men are just not father material (see chap. 6). Some men are not even worth inviting into the child's life. She needs to consider the influence he will have on her life and the child's.

There are a few types of men who may not want to be actively involved with fathering. These should be avoided:

A "No Good" Man: This guy is a loser. He is irresponsible, perhaps even criminal. As a role model for the child, he is not a good candidate.

An "Unavailable" Man: This man is a traveling type of guy. He may be a sports figure, a member of a rock group, or in general a "swinger." He probably would have difficulty remembering the name of the child, let alone be supportive.

A Married Man: His heart belongs to his wife and kids. After all, he has known her twenty years longer than you. How could he leave her and his innocent children for your child? Remember now, he told you he loved you, but that was before you got pregnant.

An Uninvolved Man: He got involved once, and that is how you got pregnant. Although he lives in town and you see him every day, he has a life to live and is not ready for fatherhood.

The "Okay, I'll Marry You" Man: He is a man of moral obligation, but he has no real interest in you and even less in "your" baby. Besides, how can he be sure that it is his child? After all, if you had sex with him, maybe you were with someone else as well.

## FATHERS WITH LIMITED ROLES

If the choice is to have the child's father in your life, what exactly will that involve? To what extent does this mean involvement between you as a couple? Are there advantages to having him involved without marriage? Limitations can be set and a cooperative relationship may be obtainable.

Support can come in many ways. Emotional support from the child's father and family may be a possibility. Grandparents of the child, with an understanding and acceptance of the situation, could be very helpful. They would have to be very special people.

Some grandparents are now receiving visitation rights with their grandchildren. But it may be difficult for them to remain open-minded and objective when it comes to "their son's child." Beware of these complications for the sake of the child. Just as divorce and custody battles can be ruthless, so can paternity involvement.

Whether he chooses to be emotionally supportive or not, the father may be responsible for the child's financial support. It may seem like a futile task to seek financial support from a disinterested party. Perhaps it is for the best. Some men are best left out of the paternal picture altogether.

The legalities of child support vary from state to state. The best way to approach this is through an attorney or child welfare agency. State laws require both parents of a child to be financially responsible for their needs. Parents may make a private agreement that can be enforced by the court. Child support awards, however, usually are lower than the true cost of raising a child.

Never-married women receive the least child support, averaging $980 a year, which is easily consumed by child care costs. The amount of support awarded may not take into account your child's special needs.

Enforcement of child support remains the task of each state. In 1984, Congress passed the 1984 Child Support Enforcement Act. In states where it is implemented, there has been an increase in cooperation from fathers.

Some judges dedicated to enforcing child support have "Pay or Stay Days." Negligent fathers are ordered to come to court with their wallets and toothbrushes. Studies show that a father's willingness to pay and ability to pay are not necessarily related. Success in receiving child support will depend on two important factors: (1) the state in which the woman resides, and (2) the judge who hears the case.

## YOUR FATHER WAS IN BANKING

Some women may want to become mothers without any relationship with a man—in any role. They may be financially sound and secure, having achieved their career goals. They realize that a husband or boyfriend does not really fit into their plans. Motherhood does, however, so they purposely pursue it.

Movies have portrayed the beautiful, successful executive who is searching for the perfect man to father her child. As it usually turns out, she is unable to separate her desire for motherhood and feelings for the man she has chosen. In the usual Hollywood fashion, it is a merry mix-up, and they all three, baby included, live happily ever after.

Fortunately for the woman serious about this choice in parenthood, there are sperm banks, which provide the needed factor for conception—sperm. Artificial insemination by donor, or AID, involves the insemination of a woman by an anonymous donor. The donor is required to provide his medical history, and his physical characteristics are recorded. (See chap. 13.)

The woman must be ovulating to become pregnant. Her responsibility is to monitor her cycle and predict ovulation. She then is inseminated by a physician who specializes in artificial insemination. She, too, will receive a questionnaire to fill out, perhaps including her motivation for wanting to become pregnant.

About 50 percent of pregnancies will occur within two months with AID. It may be necessary to repeat the insemination a few times before conception occurs.

If a woman wants to forgo insemination through a sperm bank donor, she may decide to impregnate herself with donor sperm. The donor can be a friend or an anonymous donor known only to a friend of the woman. The fertile man can masturbate and ejaculate into a sterilized jar, one that has been boiled and cooled. By using a needleless syringe, the woman draws the semen into the syringe. She then inserts the syringe deep into her vagina, as close to the cervix as she can. Lying on her back with her hips propped up by pillows, she squirts the semen in. She should remain on her back for at least half an hour. This should be repeated two to three days around ovulation time. If, after six cycles, pregnancy has not occurred, it may be necessary to consult a physician.

There are advantages as well as drawbacks to either inseminating yourself or using a sperm bank. While the donors at the sperm bank are screened, this may not be foolproof. Sperm donors receive from $25 to $40 per ejaculation. They could easily lie on their health and history forms for the money. So, in reality, there may not be much more protection through a bank than in finding a donor yourself.

If it is important to know the complete background on the donor, then you may get more than you bargained for. If you know him personally, it may be inevitable that he becomes involved in your life. This can lead to emotional and legal complications. What if he decides he wants visitation rights? Maybe he would want to give the child his last name. By being familiar with the donor, you risk the same complications as other single mothers.

If you do decide to go with donor anonymity, what do you tell your child when he asks about Daddy? The desire of adopted children to learn who their biological parents are is very strong. Would the child of a donor feel the same strong need? This child would probably spend time wondering who his father was. Knowing that there is a record somewhere, containing that information, may be difficult to live with.

Legalities such as legitimacy, financial obligations, and visitation rights become important issues. Involvement of a lawyer may be a costly move but well worth it. The definition of legitimacy varies from state to state, with some states considering children conceived by donor insemination as illegitimate. Courts may not uphold private contracts between the donor and the woman. Steps should be taken to protect the child's rights first.

The woman choosing donor insemination (DI) has many things to take into account. Not only does single parenting hold unique challenges but the gray areas of donor insemination may complicate her life as well. It is not enough to want this baby so very much. Before making this decision, a woman may want to meet and talk to other women who have experienced DI. It may be helpful to consult a child psychologist to determine what some of the effects could be on a child. It is a decision that needs careful consideration to assure a healthy, happy start for this new little person.

## BREADWINNER AND MOM: DOING IT ALL

Single motherhood involves hard work in and out of the home. Financial support may not come from the child's father. It is important to consider the implications of being single, a mother, and an employee. Before conception is the time to think about it.

More than 80 percent of single mothers work full-time, including 75 percent of those with children under six years of age. It is an asset to work where the single mother is supported; for example, medical and dental plans should cover children as well, and having a child should not influence your chances for advancement.

Probably the biggest concern of single moms is child care. A study by the U.S. House of Representatives Ways and Means Committee cites the average range of $2,000 to more than $6,500 per year for child care. This penalizes the single mother who struggles to work to make ends meet. Low-income mothers may be eligible for government assistance with child care costs. Deciding on the type of child care that is practical and economical is important.

Choosing the type of day care arrangements that work for you is important. Child care available includes day care centers, state-approved homes, non-state-approved homes, in-home care givers, and baby-sitting cooperatives.

The type of day care available and the advantages and disadvantages are as follows.

## Day Care Centers

Advantages:

- State-approved standards and requirements.
- Care givers are educated in childhood development.
- For an only child, it gives socialization.

Disadvantages:

- Center may be crowded.
- There may be a waiting list.
- More frequent illnesses.

## Private Home Providers

Advantages:

- Limited number of children on premises.
- More individualized care.
- More flexibility if mother's work hours are nontraditional.

Disadvantages:

- There are no state requirements.
- Family pets may roam freely in home, which could be a problem for child with allergies.
- Provider may stop care giving for vacation, illness, or personal reasons.

## In-Home Sitter

Advantages:

- Your child is the only one being cared for.
- The child has access to his own crib, toys, etc.
- The care is tailored to your child's needs.

Disadvantages:
- The cost is high.
- Mother must trust provider to be in the home.
- If provider is unable to make it, mother must make other arrangements.

## Baby-Sitting Cooperative
Advantages:
- A select group of mothers trades time for time.
- The women know each other.
- Minimal or no cost.

Disadvantages:
- Usually only works for part-time employed mothers.
- Must make time to pay back time you use.
- Other mothers may be busy when you need them.

## Relative (Mother, Sister, Aunts)
Advantages:
- Child knows sitter and trusts her.
- More personal investment by sitter to child's care.
- Minimal or no cost.

Disadvantages:
- Family may try to raise child "their way" if done out of charity.
- If no money is exchanged, it is difficult to debate their choice in child rearing.
- Family may tend to interfere with your personal list (work hours, job choice, friends, men).

When considering child care, become a private detective and investigate all aspects of your choice. There are a few serious considerations:

1. Safety of the environment. Toys should be age appropriate and intact. If there are pets, are they free to roam where the child is? What about pet hygiene? Are there adequate sanitary facilities for the children and care givers?

2. Your impressions of the care provider. Go to the center or home, or have the in-home sitter who will sit in your home come for an interview. Repeat these interviews if possible. Tune into the mannerisms and sensitivity of the care provider.

3. References. Even a child care center should be able to supply a list of parents currently utilizing the center's services. While there for an interview, perhaps you could meet a parent who arrives to pick up a child and briefly get an opinion.

The private sitter should be able to provide you with names of previous employers. Day care providers in private homes also should be able to supply names of other parents whom you could contact.

4. Requirements of state-approved and licensed centers and homes. These facilities have certain requirements to maintain their status. One area to consider is staff-to-child ratio. Are there more children than the care givers can handle? With the addition of infants, there should be more staff members. As many as 80 percent of children are cared for in settings that are unlicensed and unregulated. If they are state-approved and allow their standards to falter, you may have some leverage in demanding better care for your child.

5. Proximity of provider to work. For breast-feeding mothers, a quick trip to the center for feeding may be feasible. Also, mothers can join their children for lunch. If illness occurs, closer to the center is better.

6. Visitation. As the parent, you should be permitted to visit anytime. If the provider seems hesitant, be sure to pursue the reluctance with questions. The center should know who is authorized to pick up the child.

7. Illness policy. It must be understood that where there are many children, there is an increase in sickness. Most centers have policies concerning illness. Some will provide care for the sick child, while others prefer not to.

8. Values of the provider. Investigate the care provider's views on discipline and education as well as activities, group versus individual.

9. Nutrition. What types of snacks or meals are provided? Are they nutritionally sound and suited for your child? Is the food prepared under sanitary conditions? Do the providers respect your views on nutrition for your child?

10. Cost of provider. Rates will vary from one geographic location to another. Charges at large day care centers will tend to be lower, while a private in-home sitter will be the most costly. Cost may not include meals and overtime for late pickup of the child.

## NOT ALONE: MOMS NETWORKING

With the increase in never-married mothers has come increased awareness and understanding. Support groups such as Single Mothers by
Choice (SMC) have been established. SMC is a national organization
founded in 1981 and based in New York City which provides support to
single mothers and those considering single motherhood. It offers information on fertility specialists, names of sperm banks, supportive physicians, and adoption resources and holds workshops and provides support groups.

SMC encourages careful consideration when deciding on single
motherhood. The women whom they counsel tend to be in their thirties,
educated, and with a well-established career. They have weighed the
pros and cons and are willing to take on the challenge. They understand
there may be social stigmas and perhaps even work-related conflicts.
Nonetheless, their children are wanted and welcomed.

Parents Without Partners (PWP) is the largest national organization
of self-help and support for single parents. In existence for twenty-seven
years, it is a nonprofit organization for separated, divorced, never married, and widowed people who are raising kids alone. This organization
also operates internationally.

Acceptance, support, and opportunities are available for those
choosing single motherhood, which still remains the more difficult road
to travel in pursuit of parenthood. The choice to become pregnant or
remain pregnant needs to be carefully made. Weighing the pros and cons
of what life would be like with a child, on your own, is the first step.
Meeting and talking to other women who have experienced single
motherhood is advised. No one can really tell it like it is better than a
single mother, making it alone.


## SUGGESTED READING

*And Baby Makes Two*
Sharyne Meritt and Linda Steiner
Franklin Watts, 1984

*Mothers Alone*
Shelia B. Kamerman and Alfred J. Kahn
Auburn House Publishing Co., 1988

*Women as Single Parents*
Edited by Elizabeth A. Mulioy
Auburn House Publishing Co., 1988

*Who's Minding the Children?*
Margaret O'Brien Steinfels
Simon and Schuster, 1973

*Who Will Raise the Children*
James Levine
Lippincott Co., 1976

*New Conceptions*
Lori B. Andrews, J.D.
St. Martin's Press, 1984

*Begotten or Made*
Oliver O'Donovan
Clarendon Press, 1984

*Having Your Baby by Donor Insemination*
Elizabeth Noble
Houghton Mifflin Co., 1987

*The Artificial Family*
R. Snowden and G.D. Mitchell
George Allen and Unwin Ltd., 1981

*The Day Care Book*
Vicki Breithart
Alfred A. Knopf, Inc., 1974

*Ourselves and Our Children*
Boston Women's Health Book Collective
Random House, Inc., 1978

## RESOURCE GROUPS

Child Care Action Campaign
99 Hudson Street, Room 1233
New York, NY 10013
212-334-9595

Day Care Council of America
1602 17th Street, N.W.
Washington, D.C. 20036

National Association for the Education of Young Children
1834 Connecticut Avenue, N.W.
Washington, D.C. 20009
202-232-8777

"Finding Good Child Care"
Send business-size SASE to:
Checklist
Child Care Action Campaign
99 Hudson Street, Room 1233
New York, NY 10013

Children's Defense Fund
122 C Street, N.W.
Washington, D.C. 20001
202-628-8787

Parents Without Partners, Inc.
8807 Colesville Road
Silver Spring, MD 20910
301-588-9354

Single Mothers by Choice, Inc.
200 E. 84th Street
New York, NY
212-988-0993

CHAPTER 9

# SIBLINGS AND THE GOOD NEWS

*"Be gentle with the young."*

—Juvenal

## A REPEAT PERFORMANCE

Just when you and your partner get a handle on parenthood with one child, you decide to do it again. Couples in the United States space their children an average of two to four years apart. Some couples believe children should be close in age. Others prefer to have their first child in school before beginning again.

Probably the greatest concern of most parents is how the first child will accept a new sibling. Parents worry over how they will divide their time equally and what life will be like with a new baby. Concerns may surface about finances, time for themselves, and having less flexibility.

In the beginning, it is hard work to juggle a new baby and a toddler or preschooler, but it can be done. Some basic understanding of children will make the transition for the older child both smooth and exciting.

## CHILD TO CHILD

Children go through physical and developmental changes all through their young years. As parents, we have the privilege of observing their physical changes and accomplishments, but their psychological changes are not always readily apparent.

It is not always possible for children to verbalize what they are feeling, but they will let you know, somehow. What you might interpret as acting out or hostility could be their own frustrations and fears come to life.

Fortunately, the experts in child development have been able to interpret what children may be feeling at certain ages. With an understanding of what they may be thinking and feeling, we as parents can appreciate their concerns and gently guide them into becoming big brothers and sisters.

Some information on what children are experiencing in their growing minds, and how we can better help them, is presented below.

| Age | What They Are Like |
|---|---|
| *18 months* | They can say more than twenty words. |
| | They know the difference between now and later. |
| | They begin to understand separateness of themselves and others. |
| | They can open doors and undress themselves. |
| | They understand object permanence. Even if they cannot see something, they know it still exists. |
| | They may be ready to consider toilet training; if not, go easy, they still need to learn how to willingly release urine and bowel movements. They need to be approached positively. |
| *2 years* ("*terrible twos*") | They are ambivalent about their own feelings. |
| | They feel opposite to parents' feelings on many issues. |
| | This is often a stormy time. |
| | Need to be told feelings are OK. |
| *3 years* | They may have mastered the potty, girls usually before boys. |
| | They can dress and undress. |
| | They can understand longer explanations. |
| | They learn more about compromise and sharing with other children. |
| | They understand time better and know the difference between yesterday and tomorrow. |
| | They ask a lot of questions. |
| | They are adventurous and eager to explore. |
| | They become aware of sexual differences and interested in where babies come from. |
| | Many stereotypical roles are developed at this time. |
| *4 years* | They develop an expanded imagination. |
| | They may have imaginary friends. |
| | They may have nightmares about losing control. |

Parents need to reassure them that they are there to keep that from happening.

They may experiment with different personality traits.

Girls may be bolder in their play, boys may try nurturing.

They experiment with expressing various feelings.

| | |
|---|---|
| *5 and 6 years* | They begin to separate reality from fantasy. |
| | They develop memory and problem-solving skills. |
| | They learn more about the world outside of the home. |
| | They want to be older. |
| | They like to learn and make things. |
| | They have competitive influences at school. |
| | They ask questions to get answers. |
| *7 and 8 years* | Their attention span is longer. |
| | They take in knowledge through all of their senses. |
| | They learn how to seek information through books and by asking questions. |
| | They can identify feelings like anger, joy, fear. |
| | They can learn to resolve conflicts themselves. |
| | They begin to become involved in group experiences like clubs and scouts. |
| | They may begin to find loopholes in parental logic. |
| | They begin to use the phrase, "But everyone else does it." |
| *9 years* | Their perception of self broadens. |
| | They recognize their own capabilities and accomplishments and can compare them to what they could do earlier. |
| | They can commit to having responsibilities. |
| | They like rules and rely on them. |
| | They like to cooperate in group activities like 4-H and Little League. |
| | They are better organized and self-disciplined. |

They learn to lead and to follow.

*10 years* Preadolescent boys and girls separate sex with
activities like jump rope for girls, football for boys.
Girls may develop into tomboys.
They need detailed explanations on issues.
They may argue points. They need to know that it
is OK to debate and reason through an issue.
Girls may begin to develop sexually.

*11 and 12 years* Bodies are changing and feelings are out of con-
trol; girls develop an average of two years sooner
than boys.
They are learning to become adults.
They like to test their adult thinking.
They examine values outside of the family.
They feel at odds with the world, especially
authority figures, like parents.
They are sorting out who they are.
They are developing trust or distrust for other people.
They may give serious thought to education and
careers.

**Age** **How to Help Them**
*18 months* If potty training does not work, don't worry. By
getting aggravated, you lose, and so does your
baby.
Avoid using words like "Don't" and "No" when
making requests.
Explain you will be going to the hospital to have
the baby but that you will be back.
Praise them for their separateness from you.

*2 years* Do not make them suppress feelings but rather
understand and help them to redirect them.
Remind them that you accept them.
If they are not sure how they feel about the baby,
reinforce your acceptance with lots of love, hugs,
and kisses.

114

Tell them you will be available to help them with
problems, but not always to solve them.
Encourage them to verbalize their feelings.

*3 years*
Answer questions about how pregnancy occurs
honestly, in terms they can understand.
Birth of the baby can be considered a holiday, with
preparations and excitement associated with it, just
like Christmas.
When they ask when the baby is coming, try to
explain in a time frame they can grasp.

*4 years*
Encourage their imagination.
It is a good idea for boys to see father nurture the
new baby.
No need to feel threatened if when they role play
mommy or daddy, they are different from you or
your partner.
They can help you, but avoid pushing how big and
responsible they are.

*5 and 6
years*
Take time to help them learn and make things.
Answer questions openly and honestly on pregnancy, birth, breast-feeding, and the baby. This
is a wonderful time to educate them about the
wonder of new life, in a healthy, informative
manner.
They still need reassurance that you love and will
care for them.

*7 and 8
years*
You can teach about the baby by allowing them to
use their senses and experience this new little person. Allow them to explore their feelings about the
baby. Accept what they say and help them work
through their thoughts.
Continue to acknowledge their growth at a time
when the baby is the center of attention.

| | |
|---|---|
| *9 years* | Praise their accomplishments; do not allow your time with the baby to overshadow their continuing development and growth. Encourage them to be responsible for their own belongings, like their toys, room, and bike. |
| *10 years* | Encourage boys to nurture at a time when they are developing sex roles. Do not be tempted to drop the big responsibility of a baby into a child's lap. Try to recognize their need to break away. |
| *11 and 12 years* | Tune into the difficult transition into adolescence. It may be difficult for parents, but it is necessary to respect preadolescent changes, which can be quite stormy. Always remind them of your love and acceptance of them, just the way they are. |

## CHILDREN AND PREGNANCY

With an understanding of how each child perceives things at different ages, it should be easier to explain the good news. The first consideration is how soon to tell your children about the pregnancy. Telling a toddler about a new baby when you are only six weeks pregnant may mean unnecessary months of badgering. Time comprehension is important when springing the good news. When you begin to show, around the fourth or fifth month, it may be a more visible confirmation for the child.

Pregnancy lends itself to being a great opportunity for questions of exactly how babies are made. Children have a very innocent curiosity that can be used to advantage. By explaining to the child, in correct terminology and with the aid of pictures, you will satisfy their curiosity and properly inform them. Even if your child is old enough to read a book on babies by himself, always approach the subject with sensitivity. Do not just hand him a book and walk away. Follow up their reading and learning with a discussion to be sure they understand.

The age of the child may determine how involved you want them to be in the pregnancy, labor, and delivery. Some mothers are deciding to involve their children in every aspect, creating a family-centered event. You must decide what you feel is best for your child. By all means, consult the child who is old enough to understand what the process may entail. If he chooses not to be present, then respect his decision.

Consult your prenatal care giver about her policies concerning the presence of children at the delivery. Not all hospitals will accommodate siblings at the time of delivery. Home births are probably your best bet for deciding who attends the birth. Shop around for a care giver and hospital that will accommodate your preferences.

You may think you understand how your child will react to labor and delivery. Developmentally, they may seem the right age and maturity. But how do you help them through the process? The child will need a support person present just for her.

There are important considerations. Would your child be comfortable seeing you in pain, perhaps crying out on occasion? Would he be able to understand that the blood and fluids are normal? A lot of preparation should go into educating your child before the experience of labor and delivery.

Some hospitals offer sibling classes for kids. The participants visit rooms in the maternity unit and the nursery, and get some hands-on experience with dolls. The children are encouraged to express themselves, which is not too difficult for excited preschoolers. By seeing where you will be in the hospital, they are reassured that you are OK. The telephone in your room should be pointed out as the link with your child when he is at home. If he knows he can talk to mom, it seems to ease his mind.

If you breast-feed your baby, a gentle explanation is in order for your older child. This is another opportunity to educate about the human body. When you are at home, your child may feel the need to experience the breast. Allow them to suckle to taste the milk, reminding them of how much you love them. Older siblings need reassurance when a new baby arrives. While you may feel exhausted, your child wants only to be secure and to know that you still love him.

## SLOW CHANGES

With the arrival of the first child, routines and patterns of day-to-day life even out. The child knows where he sleeps, where he eats, and may even possess a concept of timing. Put yourself in your child's shoes for a moment.

One day mom says she is going to have a baby, and you, the child, must give up your crib. Maybe it is time to move into a big bed, but maybe you do not want to. Mom says the baby is due any day now and that we must get ready. So you get kicked out of your crib, maybe out of your room. Is this what this new baby is all about? You don't like this baby already!

Children need to be prepared for these changes that directly involve them. Discussing the change well in advance and allowing for cooperation and adjustment are vital for a smooth transition. The child should be moved in and accustomed to the new bed or room long before the baby arrives. This way, you can work together to make it easier for everyone involved.

Children need to know what will happen to them when mommy and daddy go to the hospital. Arrangements should be made with someone the child knows and likes. You may be gone two to three days for a normal vaginal delivery, or longer if you have a cesarean section.

Books have been written just for kids about this blessed event. They vary in age level and approach but remain excellent tools for parents. Other couples with babies may be willing to allow your child to visit and observe. Seeing how tiny and delicate a baby really is may be the seed needed to help that big brother or sister grow into a sibling. Little children need close guidance around infants. They should not, however, be chastised for their inability to be gentle. Resentments can be developed if they are constantly being told not to be so rough or not to touch the baby.

One technique used to endear the baby to the sibling is to give the child a gift from the baby. With a new baby come many baby gifts. The older child is observant and may feel left out. Naturally, the child will feel better toward this baby who comes bearing gifts for him as well.

## BIG BROTHER, BIG SISTER: BIG ADJUSTMENT

The older child may be resentful at times. After all, she has been mom and dad's center of attention. As parents anticipating the new baby, you cannot worry or expect the worst.

Try following a few simple steps in helping the child and yourselves adjust:

1. Prepare the child with his own birth experience. Recall how excited everyone was. Pull out pictures of him as a newborn, reminding him of how important he still is.

2. Involve him in prenatal checkups. Perhaps a trip to the care giver's office to hear the baby's heartbeat, followed by a stop at his favorite restaurant, would be a special time for you both.

3. Be sure he understands what will happen. Kids just basically want to know what is going to happen to them and to you during this whole process. Explain it as often as he needs to know, reassure him that he is safe and that you will come home to him.

4. Include him in the care of the baby. For the very young child, even small tasks like bringing a clean diaper to mom is a boost to his self-esteem. The older child may want to help dress and feed the baby.

Encourage contact between the children, but do not force it. If he decides he does not want to be a helper on a particular day, that is all right. He will be continuously sorting through his feelings about the new arrival.

5. Accept negative feelings. Little people are not equipped with coping skills that adults possess. So on occasion, they throw tantrums, throw toys, or just scream. Frustrations sometimes surface in that way. Be patient with your child's negative feelings whether directed toward the baby, you, or everything in general. Reassurance through hugging, touching, and kindness will help smooth those ruffled feathers.

## DETHRONING THE FIRSTBORN

Studies have found that a person's place in the family birth order can influence him for a lifetime. One reason cited is differences in how parents treat successive children.

Firstborn children in the United States seem to be favored. Everything the first child does is a novelty, from his first step to the first case he wins in court. These children tend to be breast-fed longer and have their picture taken more often. The firstborn's baby book is complete, whereas the third or fourth kid may not even have one.

Firstborns have the advantage of being an only child with an exclusive relationship with the parents. They identify strongly with parents. They tend to be high achievers: about one-third of all lawyers, doctors, astronauts, and college professors are firstborns.

Why are such shining stars found among firstborn children? Parents expect great things from them and push them to achieve. Parents are just learning to parent with the first child. They tend to punish them more severely, reward them to a greater extent, and overprotect them.

So how does this affect the golden boy or girl who is about to be knocked off the pedestal by a new baby? It is an anxious and traumatic experience. They need to be dealt with on an individual basis. Each child is his own person. But just being the elder child does not give him an adult thinking capacity. By forcing responsibility on him prematurely, you can set him up for a lifetime of resentment.

Phrases like "You should know better" directed toward a four- or five-year-old are pointless. While children do know their limits in situations, they will at times regress and need reassurance more than reprimand. They need acceptance of who they are, whether there is a baby in the house or not.

## DOUBLE THE FUN

If you are prepared for an additional, temporary disruption, then you will be ready to add a second child to your family. As experienced parents, you may even find you are more relaxed with your newborn. The confidence you have developed from parenting will allow you to enjoy the new relationships that will develop between you and your new baby and your first child and the new baby. There will be adjustments, but there really is something to the saying that it is easier the second time around.

## SUGGESTED READING FOR KIDS

*A Baby for Max*
Kathryn Laskys and Maxwell B. Knight
MacMillan Publishers, 1987

*You Were Born on Your Very First Birthday*
Linda Girard
Whitman Publisher, 1983

*How You Were Born*
Joanna Cole
William Morrow, 1984

*The New Baby*
Fred Rogers
Putnam Publishing, 1985

*The New Baby at Your House*
Joanna Cole
Morrow Publishing, 1987

*When You Were a Baby*
Ann Jonas
Greenwill Publishing, 1982

*Before You Were Born*
Margaret Sheffield
Knopf Publishing, 1984

*I Want to Tell You about My Baby*
Roslyn Banish
Wingbow Press, 1982

*Baby Brother*
Joan Walsh Anglund
Random House, 1985

## SUGGESTED READING FOR PARENTS

*Welcoming Your Second Baby*
Vicki Lansky
Bantam Books, 1984

*Your Second Child*
J. S. Weiss
Summit Books, 1981

*Understanding Your Child from Birth to Three*
J. Church
Random House, 1973

*Toddlers and Parents*
T. Berry Brazelton, M.D.
Delacorte, 1974

*To Listen to a Child*
T. Berry Brazelton, M.D.
Addison-Wesley, 1984

*Raising Kids O.K.*
Dorothy E. Babcock, R.N., M.S., and Terry D. Keepers, Ph.D.
Avon Books, 1976

# CHAPTER 10

# CAN BABIES CLIMB THE CAREER LADDER?

*"But if God had wanted us to think with our wombs,
why did He give us a brain?"*

—Clare Boothe Luce

## DREAMS OF SUCCESS

In the 1950s, if little Janie were asked what she wanted to be when she grew up, her reply would have probably been, "I want to get married and be a mommy." Her role models were traditional wives and mothers. Television portrayed the "Beav's" mother, Mrs. Cleaver, as pert and attractive, wearing a dress and, of course, an apron. She performed traditional wife/mother tasks like cooking, cleaning, and worrying. She was content and had ambitions only to keep her windows sparkling, feed her family, and keep her freckled-faced son out of trouble.

In the 1980s, we have television heroines who are doctors, lawyers, and, yes, liberated wives and single mothers. Women have changed their goals to include education, career, and families. We have observed our predecessors and admired their dedication to motherhood. The generations before us have been women who sensed the need for careers and families and yet were not supported by the male-dominated society. If they did enter the work force, it was more out of necessity than to fulfill career goals.

Nearly half of all mothers in the United States are returning to work before their child reaches his first birthday. Mothers with children under three are now the fastest-growing group to enter the work force. However, our society has not been quick to accept these changes in our roles. Some believe that working mothers weaken the family and that if a woman wants to work, she should not have children.

These social attitudes will have to change. The fact is that women are reentering the work force after their babies are born. Employers and legislators must accept this reality and change accordingly. As long as they are not accommodating working mothers, they lose, and so do the children.

In 1987, the Act for Better Child Care Services, or "ABC bill," was introduced in the U.S. House and Senate. The promoters of the bill recognize the difficulty families have in balancing both job and family responsibilities. The bill could help in several ways. It is expected to increase the availability of child care, improve the quality of care, and make child care more affordable for lower-income families. Helping welfare mothers find and afford child care would increase their self-sufficiency, promoting a decrease in welfare needs. The program would cost the government $2.5 billion.

Sounds like a lot of money, but it is nothing compared with the $10 billion it takes to keep single mothers on welfare and out of the workplace. The government thinks nothing of spending billions of dollars on nuclear arms, cleaning up oil spills, and space exploration. Our children are, as Herbert Hoover said, "our most valuable natural resource." They should be considered a worthwhile national investment.

Meanwhile, working mothers must find ways to meet obligations to both family and job. Some couples work different shifts so that only a few hours overlap when a sitter may be necessary. For example, Kathy is a nurse and works the 11:00 p.m. to 7:00 a.m. shift at a hospital. Her husband, Ian, works 8:00 a.m. to 4:00 p.m. at a factory. While this schedule does not mean much time together, it allows them to cover the care of their son, Jimmy. Kathy gets home around 7:30 a.m., just in time to kiss Ian good-bye and try to catch an hour or two of sleep before Jimmy wakes up. When Ian gets home, Kathy goes to bed. For them it is the best arrangement that will allow them both to work and still care for their son at home.

Other women may choose to cut back from full-time to part-time work. This may correspond with using a sitter, day care, or coordinating hours with their partners' day off. Some progressive companies and businesses offer flex time to their employees. Women then can work in coordination with their child care schedule and still get their jobs accomplished.

Still other mothers decide to try working at home, as entrepreneurs. Not everyone is cut out to be a home-based businesswoman. The benefits of being with your child may be offset by the difficulty of running a business at home. To be truly successful at both, you still must be prepared for adjustments and challenges.

Child care arrangements need to be carefully coordinated around parents' jobs. It is like a triangle. Child care, mom's job, and dad's job are the three sides. Each side must be equally proportioned to create a secure working schedule. It is not even as simple as that. Parents suffer from tremendous guilt and anxiety about leaving their carefully planned, beloved baby in the hands of someone else. One question that women frequently ask themselves is, "Why did I have a child if I cannot spend time with him?"

Mothers need to remind themselves of the basic concept of quality versus quantity. The sad truth is that mothers at home with their kids full time probably do not spend any more quality time with their kids than working mothers do. Television, VCRs, play groups, and shopping malls are the entertainment children are experiencing. A mother working outside of the home looks forward to coming home and unwinding with her child snuggled close and reading a Dr. Seuss book.

Ask any father who works all day at a high-pressure job. Having a child yell, "Daddy's home!" and run to his arms is just the sedative needed. It works the same way with working mothers

Until working moms can free themselves of guilt, this aspect of career and motherhood will be unresolved. A thriving, happy child is the proof that mothers can mother and work.

## WORKING PREGNANT

What influences do jobs have on pregnancy? This question should be answered before you become pregnant. In fact, close investigation into potentially harmful situations is a responsible act on the couple's part. Chemical substances, radiation, and stress can be involved in any number of occupations.

A few guidelines for determining potentially hazardous situations are as follows:

1. Assess your work area. Are you involved with chemicals or fumes like those that might be present in hairdressing salons, mills or industrial plants, chemical plants, or dry cleaning establishments?

2. Hospital workers including laboratory technicians, X-ray technicians, and even nurses who must work with immobile patients should carefully examine their responsibilities.

3. Learn from your employer what chemicals you must handle. Find out the exact name of the chemical or toxic substance.

4. Express your concerns to your employer and ask what the policies are concerning relocation, if necessary, for the duration of the pregnancy.

5. If you are not supported by your employer, request assistance from your obstetrician in encouraging your employer to consider pregnancy a time for safety first.

6. If you are not able to reach your employer through your own efforts, contact the National Institute for Occupational Safety and Health. (See Resource Groups, below.)

7. Stress is a part of daily living but can be hazardous to your fetus if overdone. A psychological overload accompanied by fatigue places a pregnant woman at risk for a miscarriage or premature delivery. Learning to relax, using relaxation techniques, can help you cope with stress. If a high-pressure job is causing you mental anguish, give up the job or prepare yourself by learning to cope before you become pregnant.

8. Women using video display terminals may be concerned for the safety of their fetuses. While it is a worthwhile consideration, a recent study published reassuring data. The radiation level emitted by VDTs is very low, and it is believed that these low levels would not be harmful to humans or experimental animals. If this is a continued concern for you, be sure to talk to your doctor about it.

## BLUE COLLAR OR BUSINESS SUIT: THE CHALLENGE IS THERE

The first thing the working couple should do is define what benefits are available from her employer. The preconceptional couple has a right to receive information concerning maternity leave as well as paternity leave. Other areas that should be discussed are time available for leave if the pregnancy is high risk, if the baby is premature, if the baby is sick and hospitalized, and if the mother needs more than six weeks maternity leave. The couple also needs to ask about paid leave of absence, job resumption after an absence, seniority, benefits, and the possibility of job sharing if appropriate.

Pregnancy disability leave is different from maternity leave. In 1978, the Pregnancy Disability Act was passed. This is the only nationally legislated policy solely for the protection of pregnant women in the workplace. It requires that a company with fifteen or more employees include pregnancy in its list of disabilities covered. The leave is from two to ten weeks for a normal pregnancy and delivery. The time can be used before the baby is born or from the day the child is born.

Maternity leave is time above and beyond the pregnancy-related disability leave. It is individualized, based on the company's policy. The

126

larger the company, the more flexible and generous leave policies tend to be. Companies with a high proportion of women managers and executives also will lean toward a more flexible leave policy. But no woman can assume her workplace owes her either maternity leave or pregnancy disability leave. This is why it is so important to investigate company policies even before taking a job, not to mention before conception.

Another area to consider is job security with pregnancy leave. The employer who has a limited leave may not have to guarantee your job to you if you choose to remain on leave. In fact, the longer you are away, the more likely the small employer is to replace you and reinstate you somewhere else when you return.

This is a difficult decision for the pregnant woman. After all, no one can predict how the pregnancy, birth, and new parent adjustments will go. Six weeks is not a very long time to grasp parenting let alone catch up on your sleep. But you are faced with the possibility of losing the position you have worked so hard for. The pros and cons must be examined carefully.

Most women work in companies that offer no maternity benefits and live in states that have no regulated job-protected maternity leave. They are neither job-protected nor financially secure once they deliver their babies.

The United States is quite backward in its views on parental leave. The minimum paid leave offered in Western Europe is fourteen weeks, with a maximum of five months. In Finland, national maternity insurance covers men and women for six months. Sweden pays 90 percent of a parent's salary for up to nine months. Legislators have a long road ahead to meet the needs of our society. Employers must recognize the need to accommodate the women employees who manage and run their corporations, businesses, and factories.

## DIAPER BAGS AND BRIEFCASES

It is inevitable that the day will come to return to work. If there is a choice about when to return, what would be a good time? Some women are ready as soon as they have their doctor's go-ahead. Usually by six weeks, they are close to returning to their prepregnant physical state, or are they?

Going back to work requires clear thinking and stamina. Depending on your job, you may need more of one or the other. If your body is not ready, you can only do more harm to yourself. You undergo physical as well as emotional changes, both of which can be draining.

Perhaps the greatest drain to your system is sleep deprivation. The last weeks of pregnancy are not particularly restful for the woman. Her large uterus weighs on her bladder. Slumber occurs in short periods rather than a long, undisturbed night of rest. After delivery, if you are breastfeeding you will do so perhaps every two to three hours for the first several weeks. Even bottle feeding the newborn requires you or your partner to be awake perhaps two to three times during normal sleeping hours. A woman may want to delay returning to work if at all possible so that she can establish breast-feeding patterns.

The baby has a schedule to be considered as well. The first three months are vital for developing the parent-child relationship. At around four months, babies do not seem to mind being left with care givers. Between eight and twelve months, babies develop stranger anxiety. It is ill-advised to place a child with an outside care giver at this time. This may mean either doing it early, around four months, or waiting until the child is older. Actually, the earlier you return to work, when the child is around four months, the easier the separation may be for you both.

Child care is another factor in determining when you may want to return to work. If the choice is made in advance of the pregnancy or birth, this allows for time to explore possibilities. (See chap. 8 on child care.) It is vital to your peace of mind to have made your decision and believe in your choice before the baby arrives.

With some child care centers, it may be necessary to be on a waiting list. It is important that you and the care giver share the same child-rearing beliefs. These should be established before the baby is born.

Job security and monetary needs also govern timing in returning to work. If you cannot afford more than six weeks off, then you are financially obligated to return to work. If your job cannot, or will not, be promised to you if you take more leave, this, too, is an incentive to return as soon as possible.

Money can also be a reason to remain home. Some couples find child care costs to be in excess of the woman's salary. This can apply to the father's job as well, which leads some men to quit work and stay home to take care of the baby.

Personal situations govern the time to return to work, if it is necessary or desired. Employer attitudes toward parents is another area to investigate. How flexible is the system that demands a woman return to work six weeks after her baby is born?

Job sharing is an option chosen by some women. The hours, pay, and benefits of a full-time job are divided with another person. Flex-time allows the employee a chance to work forty hours and yet have some choice in starting and quitting times. This makes it easier to juggle home, family, and a full-time job.

Larger institutions like banks accommodate by having "mother hours." These hours generally are from 9:00 a.m. to 2:00 or 3:00 p.m. While some employers are trying to create easier life-styles for families, they still remain in the minority.

Returning to work requires time and patience. Scheduling begins at home with coordination. Feeding and dressing yourself and your child will require extra time in the morning. Once you make it to work, do not be surprised if thoughts of your baby keep surfacing. Of course, you will miss her and long to be with her. Guilt pangs may distract you temporarily.

The effect of a mother's employment on her child can be related to her attitude. Studies show that in groups of children with employed mothers, kids were more self-sufficient and peer oriented. Children with nonemployed mothers were more adult oriented and dependent.

To believe that children are penalized by working mothers is to deny the truth. Children are able to learn and develop special qualities in most situations. A working mother needs to work through her own guilt and attitudes in order to create a positive experience.

## RETURNING TO WORK: NECESSITY VS. LUXURY

It is clear that returning to work is necessary for some women. A decision made before the delivery of the child may have to be changed after the birth. Monetary needs should be examined carefully to determine if the cost of child care outweighs the income from the woman's job. If you desire to stay home but fear loss of income, it may be worth working on a budget.

For example, it is obvious that life-styles change after the arrival of a baby. With these changes there will naturally need to be financial adjustments. This may mean fewer luxuries and more saving for necessities. What are just typical life-style preferences to some are luxuries to others.

Another area to consider is career ladder position. If you have worked for the past ten years and made advancements in your career, do you want to stop completely? Is there a particular level you desire to achieve before you will be content? If that is the case, perhaps pregnancy should be delayed until the pinnacle is reached.

There is no guarantee that you will be able to leave your mother job to return to your career. As a working mother, you are employed in two jobs. It is difficult to give either job 100 percent of yourself. That is not to say that you will not give each your best. You have needs and so does your child. Together with your partner, you will be able to decide if your income is a necessity or an added bonus. If your job is important enough to need your immediate return after the baby's birth, then rest comfortable in your choice.

If it were possible to survive on one income and put your job on hold for a year or more, what would that involve? Assuming finances would be stable, what does it really mean to turn to motherhood as a career?

## WORK WITHDRAWAL

Although we think we know what staying home involves, it may be a bigger challenge than you realize. After all, you do not have to get up early to dress, curl your hair, put on your makeup, and make it to work by eight. Your demanding occupation will no longer drive you to tears when everything is going wrong. There will be no boss to monitor your coffee breaks or your lunch hour. No longer haunted by all the things you disliked about your job, your new job as a stay-home mother is going to be a breeze.

Motherhood is really no different from your previously held job. You will have different types of challenges. You will not need to get up early for your grooming and you probably will not care. Your sleeping patterns will change to two- to three-hour intervals. Your new boss will change size and age but will still determine whether you can relax with a cup of coffee in the morning. The biggest adjustment is not being able to leave your job after eight hours is over. Your job as a mother is twenty-four hours a day, every day, even when you are away from your family.

Falling apart and shedding tears are not unique to high-pressure jobs. Motherhood produces as much pressure as any corporate executive could ever experience. Frustrations and doubts in our capabilities as mothers take their toll on the strongest office managers.

Staying home with your child can lead to the "hazards of home life." Probably the most devastating is accessibility to the kitchen. Our kitchens are like the sirens of mythology, beckoning us to enter and partake of their bounties. We are pushed into the kitchen to prepare our children's food, make meals, and, of course, snack. Commercials on television are the catalysts that boot us out of our chairs toward the kitchen. We see the baked goods, drinks, and goodies and just have to put something in our mouths. Advertisers know exactly who the consumer is and how to get to her.

Women's magazines give us a mixed message about what we should be doing. The articles in the front are about losing weight quickly, keeping your marriage alive, and knitting your child's entire school wardrobe. The back half of the magazines are food advertisements and recipes. Once again, we are considered the goddesses of food and cooking. Beware of the advertiser's techniques for reaching the consumer. They are after us. Staying at home is a good time to tune into nutrition and diet to assure a quick and healthy recovery of your prepregnant state.

Television is still the greatest source of entertainment and information we have. The early morning news shows are professional and informative. As the day goes on, the quality of viewing diminishes. Game shows and daytime drama are great for killing time. The beneficial input from them is questionable. It may be fun at first to think about watching whatever you want during the day. If you have had a fulfilling career or job, the fun will not last. It may even turn to frustration or boredom.

That may be enough to drive you to begin calling everyone you know. Of course, most careers or jobs involve working with other people on a daily basis. Talking, sharing, and laughing together are taken for granted in the workplace. And your home with a newborn becomes a lonely, adult-free environment. Granted, there is a period when the quiet pace is appealing. Then, you notice that when your partner comes home from work, you follow him around the house, so glad to see an adult who speaks in complete sentences.

During the day you may need that same verbal communication, hence the telephone becomes your source for outside contact. The only problem is that most of your friends are working and do not have time to talk to you during the day. But they would love to see you and have lunch next Thursday. Can you make it? Oh, you are breast-feeding, guess that will not do, maybe some other time.

As it usually goes, friends without children are on a different wavelength from you. You may notice a gradual loss of contact with your friends as your interests change and your flexibility is limited. This may feel bad at first, but it is a transition into parenthood. You are growing with each transition you make.

Having established diversions before the baby is born is important. Although a lot of your time will be taken by the baby, you can use your new life-style to your advantage. Correspondence courses are available on any subject. Crafts and baking could lead to developing your own home-based business. Entrepreneurs in a variety of businesses are mothers at home. Free-lance artists, writers, and photographers can keep busy marketing from their home and still maintain their child's care. It is important to be realistic in these goals as well.

Mothering at home requires some emotional adjustments:

- Whatever your family income, work within its limits. Life-style changes are difficult but are worth the struggle in the long run.
- Babies are not newborns forever. This means that they become less dependent and more rewarding as they respond to you. They do actually become pleasurable and help alleviate the sense of loss from unemployment.
- The time you spend with your child can never be replaced. You may feel burdened at times, but the fact is you can be productive as both mother and career person. By keeping your mind active, you are preparing for your return to the workplace.
- If you need more support, mothers' groups are available in your area. Participants are women who choose to stay home with their children. A well-organized group might hold educational meetings and bake sales and coordinate trips for themselves and their children.

Some hospitals with support groups are open to starting mothers' groups. The basic ingredients needed are a few interested mothers, advertisements, and backing from an organization that promotes support groups. The YWCA and women's health care centers may have information on groups in your area. Or the motivated mother may start a group of her own.

## LIKE PICKLES IN VINEGAR: CAREERS KEEP

In this dog-eat-dog world, career women are driven like their male counterparts to succeed. In fact, they may have to be better to be treated equally. Even with all the blood, sweat, and tears experienced by women in the work force full time, they still only make the equivalent of 70 cents for each dollar a man makes.

We feel the need to pursue careers. We also feel the need to become mothers. So which job deserves 100 percent of our energy? Neither. Careers and motherhood both tend to be overrated. In fact, they can actually enhance each other. We need to become more confident that we can handle both, or either, as we choose. Stay-home mothers and career mothers have been disagreeing over which choice is right for years. We need to support each other and achieve a balance in our individual lives.

Giving 100 percent to both job and mothering can never happen. Instead, by giving your best to each, or either, you will be able to achieve realistic goals. When we learn to accept our capabilities and believe that our choices on working and mothering are right for us, then both become enjoyable experiences.

## SUGGESTED READING

*The Working Parents Survival Guide*
S. W. Olds
Bantam Books, 1983

*Pregnant While You Work*
Wenda Morrone
Macmllan, 1984

*The Working Woman Report*
Editors of Working Woman, with Gay Bryand
Simon and Schuster, 1984

*Time Out for Motherhood*
Lucy Scott and Merideth Joan Angwin
Jeremy P. Tarcher, Inc., 1986

*Monday Through Friday: Daycare Alternatives*
Jane Merrill Filstrup
Teachers College Press, 1982

*Managing Your Maternity Leave*
Meg Wheatly and Marcie Hirsch Schorr
Houghton Mifflin, 1983

*Can Babies Climb the Career Ladder?*

*Working and Caring*
T. Berry Brazelton, M.D.
Addison-Wesley, 1985

*The Crisis of the Working Mother:*
*Resolving the Conflict Between Family and Work*
Barbara J. Berg, Ph.D.
Summit Books, 1986

*Pregnancy and Working*
Jean Grasso Fitzpatrick
Avon Books, 1984

*Maternity Policies and Working Women*
Alfred J. Kahn and Paul Kingston
Columbia University Press, 1983

*Working Pregnant*
Jane Hughes Paulson
Fawcett Columbine, 1984

## RESOURCE GROUPS

Child Care Action Campaign
99 Hudson Street, Room 1233
New York, NY 10013
212-334-9595

Day Care Council of America
1602 17th Street, N.W.
Washington, D.C. 20063

National Association for the
Education of Young Children
1834 Connecticut Avenue, N.W.
Washington, D.C. 20009
202-232-8777

Child Care Handbook
To Order: Children's Defense Fund
122 C Street, N.W.
Washington, D.C. 20001


The Women's Occupational Health Resource Center
117 St. John's Place
Brooklyn, NY 11217
718-230-8822
Self-addressed, stamped envelope for a free list of publications.


National Institute for Occupational Safety and Health Publications R-6
4676 Columbia Parkway
Cincinnati, OH 45226
513-533-8236


National Commission on Working Women
2000 P Street, N.W.
Suite 508
Washington, D.C. 20036
202-737-5764


The National Council on the Future of Women in the Workplace
c/o The National Federation of Business and Professional Women's
Clubs, Inc.
2012 Massachusetts Avenue, N.W.
Washington, D.C. 20036
202-293-1100


9 to 5, the National Association of Working Women
1224 Huron Road
Cleveland, OH 44115


Women's Legal Defense Fund
2000 P Street N.W.
Washington, D.C. 20036
202-887-0364

National Alliance of Home-based Business Women
P.O. Box 95
Norwood, NJ 07648

Women Entrepreneurs
3061 Fillmore Street
San Francisco, CA 94123
415-929-0129

The Child Care Resource Center
187 Hampshire Street
Cambridge, MA 02139
617-547-9861

Day Care and Child Development Council of America
1012 14th Street, N.W.
Washington, D.C. 20005

CHAPTER 11

# MONEY
## The Root of All Families

*"Money doesn't always bring happiness. People with ten million dollars*
*are no happier than people with nine million dollars."*

—Hobart Brown

## INCOMES AND OUTCOMES

In the United States, we can have a television in every room, a driveway
full of cars, and prime rib in every pot. There is no doubt that the average U.S. citizen is probably quite comfortable, or is he?

Have we sacrificed our time for money and our money for time?
Money is what we must have to survive, and yet it is still an elusive goal
to be economically sound and comfortable. Understanding the basics of
money will enable you and your partner to plan for a secure, yet enjoyable future.

Income will always influence the outcome of financial security.
Security versus luxury is an issue worth examining. The couple with two
incomes and no children can probably count on a comfortable existence.
When considering parenthood, however, advance planning is needed.

Many families require two incomes to pay the bills and still put food
on the table. What it amounts to is working with the income you have to
meet needs. Relying on two incomes too heavily may lead to unexpected
complications.

Chris and Bonnie were a dual income couple. They each had a
yearly income of about $20,000. They had worked for ten years before
they decided to have a child. Bonnie had a history of heart problems and
was advised to quit work and remain home the last three months of her
pregnancy. That did not present a problem for Chris and Bonnie, at first.

Bonnie was able to draw on her parental leave before the birth of
their child. She planned to return to work six weeks after the baby was
born. What they did not count on was a complicated delivery.

Bonnie had to remain off work for three months. Not only did she
not receive a paycheck but she also needed help with the baby. Family
was not an option for help, because they lived in another state. They had

to employ a nurse to help Bonnie and care for the child. What used to be a comfortable economic situation was now a strain on their new family. Planning for unexpected expenses is an option that could have helped Chris and Bonnie budget better.

Lou and Marian lived modestly on Lou's income for five years. They planned two years earlier to begin a family and started a savings account. The "baby" account consisted of twenty dollars a week out of Lou's income. They promised each other to keep the account solely for unexpected needs for the baby. They conceived and delivered their son right on schedule.

Not concerned with designer baby clothes and furniture, Marian bought used baby clothes and borrowed a crib, high chair, and changing table from a friend. They were accustomed to working within their budget and planned to continue. Planning by opening a savings account for the baby was just that added security they felt was right for them.

One-income families are advised to keep six months worth of living expenses in a savings account for emergency purposes. Insurance policies should be updated: a life insurance policy should provide 75 percent of the breadwinner's wages to the family. The woman working at home should also be covered with a small term policy as well as a retirement fund. Most important, both partners should know what their policies cover and what the terms are for any financial investments.

Dual-career families must first learn to set priorities in spending and be willing to eliminate extras. They must think about child care costs, which can range from $1,500 to $10,000 annually, with the average amount of day care costing around $3,000 a year. The two-income family can choose the best benefits from employment packages and combine them to have the most complete coverage.

In either case, economic planning for the addition of a child is a wise decision and can prevent financial disasters. It is important for both members of this parental partnership to understand money and how to handle it. Even in traditional one-income families, where the man handles the finances, a woman needs to have an equal understanding and voice in money matters. Planning may include learning to sacrifice and compromise life-style for financial security.

## HOW COULD A SMALL KID COST SO MUCH?

Babies are so small and helpless at birth. It is hard to believe they could ever cost much to feed and clothe. The fact is they cost thousands of dollars even before they are born. It is important to have complete medical coverage with top-of-the-line maternity benefits.

Once conception has occurred, a woman should seek prenatal care. Prenatal visits to a private obstetrician, including any testing that may be ordered, are usually covered by insurance. It is important to know what your health care coverage includes before conceiving. Once you are pregnant, it is not probable that you will be able to secure maternity benefits or increase the coverage you have. Prenatal visits will vary in cost according to your location and, of course, your care giver's area of specialization. Prenatal clinics help women by adjusting their fees on a sliding scale.

A normal vaginal delivery and two- to three-day hospital stay may average from $2,500 to $3,000 for mother and baby. The trend for women to be discharged within twenty-four hours after birth may help shorten hospitalization.

If a woman has a cesarean section, there is the additional cost of the operating room. Since it is considered major surgery, it could mean an average of $3,500 to $4,000 for the mother's bill. The baby, without any complications, would be an additional $1,000 to $1,500. Average hospital stays for cesarean births are usually around five days.

Once the baby is delivered, he starts his own hospital tab, just by staying in the nursery. Any testing, like blood work, and supplies, like diapers and formula, are included in his price tag. Your insurance will cover all these items.

If you choose to have your male child circumcised, as of now, you will pay for it out of your own pocket. The payment status of this procedure may change again in the future. Be sure to discuss that decision carefully before the baby is born. The baby's bill is included with yours as the total shown on your insurance statement.

The baby will have to be seen by either a pediatrician or your family doctor while in the hospital. You should decide before delivery who you want and make this known on admission to the hospital. This will add another charge to the bill. Finding out what the baby's doctor charges before the delivery and for well baby checkups may be necessary.

Babies need frequent and regular checkups during the first years of life. They are checked for their development and given immunization shots. It is worthwhile finding a doctor who is current on children's health and with whom you can discuss your concerns. If he is affordable as well, you have found a gem.

Consideration of the cost of a child before conception may help you plan your budget more realistically. It makes sense that the older children become, the more expensive they are. Their basic needs of food, clothing, and accessories increase.

Hand-me-down clothes from relatives and friends are probably realistic for everyday clothes and casual attire. Investment in those cute little outfits may backfire. In the first year, babies grow so fast that if you buy a pink ruffled dress with matching bonnet and booties for $25, you better put it on her every day to get your money's worth.

Well, you say, we'll just save it for the next child, when this one outgrows it. You can do that if the next two kids are also girls; otherwise you may be sorry you invested so heavily.

The pregnant woman also outgrows her clothes. With the changes occurring in pregnancy, your body will need a new wardrobe. Women seem to have a wonderful camaraderie when it comes to lending each other maternity clothes. Let's face it, you only wear these clothes for about six months, so who wants to pay a fortune for a temporary new look? It is an added expenditure at a time when you are trying to desperately cut back.

Sensible clothes buying should be part of your financial adjustments. Let friends and family buy you or your little one something special to wear. People enjoy doing something special for mothers and babies-to-be.

To help you understand what you are in for as parents, it may be of benefit to see how and when your child spends your money. In 1982, according to the U.S. Department of Agriculture, the cost of raising a child to the age of 18 was about $134,414. This does not include the cost of college. The first five years are not too bad. Most of this money is spent on housing and food, with clothing close behind.

After a child starts school, costs increase. Approximately 40 percent of the total cost is utilized when children are between 12 and 17 years of age. Their needs and luxuries cost more. You must keep growing teens in clothes and shoes for both school and play. Because our children are members of the high-tech generation, a checkerboard just will not do when video games are available.

Because the larger part of their expenses occurs when they are teens, you will have a chance to begin budgeting and saving for the expensive years. Preparing before they are born, by budgeting and beginning that special savings account, will allow you more time to save.

It may seem cold and calculated to itemize the costs of a child. After all, it is a human life that can have no price tag. However, understanding what lies ahead will help the you and your partner plan for a secure economic future.

## THE ROOF OVER YOUR HEAD

"Darling, I'm pregnant. Are you happy? Are you surprised? What will our families say, our friends, our landlord?"

"I am happy, dear, and our friends and family will be, too. The landlord, I fear, will not."

A situation not unusual for couples who live in apartments is the possibility of outgrowing their home. When signing a lease, you and your partner should be sure children are welcome in your apartment complex. Some places welcome neither kids nor pets. If conception occurs and you are still under lease, you may have to find a new place to live. Planning a pregnancy is beneficial to avoid having to make snap decisions about housing.

If time allows, it may benefit you to compare renting versus buying a home. Your job, income, location, and future plans will determine whether you still want to rent or buy your home. There are advantages and disadvantages to both. An important point to remember is that it must fit into your budget present and future. As difficult as it may sound, it may be necessary to project into your future to help you decide what is the right choice for you.

## WHAT ABOUT WHEELS?

You and your partner look good driving around in that 1974 MGB. The top is down, the cherry red paint is glistening in the sun, and the black interior is in mint condition. What a classic, what a beauty. Where will you put the car seat for the baby? Oh, well. It is time to think about practical transportation.

Cars are probably the second most important investment you will have to make. Perhaps more practical considerations should be made when considering this purchase for the family-to-be.

Your financial status and credit rating will be taken into account when you go to a financial lending institution for a loan. Once style and speed may have been determining factors in car buying. For most people considering the family life-style, reliability, size, and cost of maintenance are determining factors in the purchase of a vehicle.

## INSURED TO DEATH

We need it, we have to have it, but how much is too much? To drive a car, you are required to have insurance coverage that includes property damage and liability. You are required to have homeowner's insurance to secure a mortgage; sometimes the borrower is even required to have life insurance.

While medical insurance is not required by law, it is the only way to handle the high cost of health care. Life insurance policies are a security meant for the survivors of the policy holder. This type of insurance should be considered by anyone who has children. Each type of insurance can be easily understood if explained in uncomplicated terms.

### Automobile Insurance

We all know how important our car is in our lives. Without vehicles we are a paralyzed society. And yet, the car is both a weapon and a way of life. Liability coverage protects you, the car owner, from claims brought by property owners, pedestrians, or other drivers who say you are at fault. Other parts of car insurance anatomy include uninsured motorist coverage, collision and comprehensive coverage, and possibly personal injury protection.

Compare coverage and costs with other agencies for the best deal for you. Be sure to ask about discounts that may decrease your premium cost. For example, a female driver between 30 and 64 years of age who is the only driver of her car can receive a five to ten percent discount. A car pool participant can receive anywhere from a ten to twenty percent discount. Do not let agents pressure you into buying more insurance than you can afford or than your car is worth.

### Home Owner's Insurance

The protection of your family home and possessions is a necessity for financial security. Nothing could be more tragic than a fire that wipes out a house and its belongings. While insurance cannot bring back the possessions that held sentimental value, a good policy can rebuild a home and allow for a new beginning.

There are basic, broad, and special coverages for home owners. With added coverage comes added cost. It is important to have enough coverage to pay for the rebuilding of your home. The age of your home, the location, and the type of construction will determine the cost of your home owner's insurance.

The average costs are anywhere from $200 to $3,000 a year. Once again, shop for the best possible coverage at an affordable price for you.

## Life Insurance

Life insurance, pure and simple, is to insure that your dependents are financially taken care of if you should die prematurely. If a person has no dependents, then he or she should have enough insurance for burial costs.

Married persons may want enough to provide their spouse with a lifetime income. Probably the most important time to secure a complete life insurance policy is when becoming a parent. You must not only meet the current financial needs of your children but their future needs as well.

There are a variety of policies available. Some include investment of the premiums, which can be borrowed against in the future. It is vital to have a policy that will cover the cost of raising a child or children and furthering their education.

But do not let yourself be talked into so much insurance that you can hardly pay the premiums. It is wise to consider the "what ifs," but be aware of your present economic state and needs as well.

## Health Insurance

Health insurance is probably one of the best investments you can make. When planning to have a child, a complete policy with sound maternity coverage is vital. Most employers offer some type of health insurance coverage.

Group policies typically pay 80 percent of the medical expenses, after a $100 deductible. This is compared to individual health policies that can range from $1,200 to $4,600 a year for a family of four. The group policy is definitely a much better deal. In the end, either policy is still better than no insurance at all.

It is extremely important to know what coverage your policy includes before you get pregnant. Prenatal testing, prenatal checkups, hospitalization, labor and delivery, and all necessary care for the baby should be included in the coverage. A complete health care coverage policy is a necessity for a growing family.

Another type of health care coverage is provided by Health Maintenance Organizations, or HMOs. Members of HMOs include a primary physician who is always seen first by the patient. He may refer you to other doctors but must always be consulted first. Pharmacists, nurses, laboratory technicians, and other doctors are all contracted by the HMO. Choice of hospitals may be limited. If you are lucky, your family doctor may be a member of an HMO as well as your local hospital.

The advantage of the HMO is that there is a fixed monthly or yearly charge to belong. This cuts down on the complication of paying deductibles and filing claims for yourself and your care giver. If your employer offers this type of coverage, look into it and be sure it meets your needs. Remember the need for complete maternity coverage.

## CAN WE BUY A BUDGET?

What seems like torture but is really an act of self-control? Give up? It is a budget.

If you do not have a budget, now is the time to begin the analysis and change. It begins by examining where the money you make goes after you receive your paycheck.

About 70 percent of your income goes to major expenses including housing and taxes and perhaps car payments and insurance. The remainder slips away almost unseen, when you buy clothes, electronic gadgets, groceries, gifts, entertainment, and, of course, when you use those plastic demons, credit cards.

Figuring out where the money goes is as simple as reading your old checks, receipts, and credit card statements. It is a good idea to sit down and list all expenditures for one month. Take everything into account, down to the last cheeseburger from McDonald's. It all adds up. Taking account on paper is the first painless step toward establishing a budget.

The next step is to decide where to cut the expenses. One of the first places to start is cutting back use of credit cards, unless it is a dire necessity. The luxury awarded you by the use of that plastic card can cost you as much as 18 percent in interest annually. Each time you carry payments over from month to month, you are charged interest. So be sure to think twice before you say, "Charge it."

Now you know where the extra money is going, and now you must redirect it. As was mentioned before, babies just naturally become more expensive. The expense of a child must be incorporated into the budget in a realistic manner. One way to appreciate the cost of a baby is to go browsing in the stores to study baby items. Jot down how much diapers, or cans of formula, cost. Then look at baby food and shoes to support those growing feet. Before you conceive is the perfect time to study the expense of a baby, assess your spending habits, and establish a new workable budget for your family.

## Long-Term Goals

With a firm budget established, you may find you have some "extra" money. Let's face it, there is no such thing as extra money but rather money that could possibly make more money for you.

It has been concluded that a savings account could be started as an emergency fund. A baby account could be started, upon conception, to be used for the baby, or by the child for college.

Retirement funds are popular forms of investment and a security for the future. Both men and women can benefit from Individual Retirement Accounts (IRAs) or Keogh accounts. It is a sound investment for the future and not really a financial drain. Consult any bank, savings and loan, credit union, brokerage, mutual fund, or insurance company for information on retirement accounts.

To send a child to college for four years will cost today's parents $18,000. Thinking about college education funding cannot be started too soon. There are educational loans, grants, and for that motivated kid, scholarships. All of these can help ease the burden.

As with any investment, you must examine current as well as future needs. While educational savings accounts are important, be realistic with how much you can afford to deposit monthly. After all, your newborn will need diapers before he needs textbooks.

## A WILL

A loving act that many people do not consider is that of making a will. When considering the creation of a new life, why should parents-to-be think about death? Well, death is part of that continuous circle of life.

What is truly tragic is for a man or woman to die without preparing for those left behind. Parenthood brings great responsibilities and the need to prepare for even the most tragic of situations. Couples should have wills that leave their estates to each other. It is wrongly assumed that if a man dies without a will, his wife would inherit his share of the estate.

If there are minors, the estate will be divided equally. If there is a $150,000 estate, and the couple has two children, the wife would receive $50,000, and each child would receive the same. Sounds simple, except that to gain access to the children's inheritance, the mother would have to go to court. The state would appoint a guardian for the children's inheritance. It can be very complicated and expensive and can be avoided by making a will.

Preparation of a will should be done by an expert. A lawyer familiar with your state laws and taxes is the best person to consult. A simple will may range from $50 to $150 for preparation. The more complicated, the more costly. Legal clinics can offer an adequate will in the price range of $50 or less.

One of the most important parts of a will is the assignment of a guardian for your children, should both parents die. Some things to consider are:

1. Age of potential guardians. If grandparents are to be the caretakers of your children, will they be able to care for young children?

2. Marital stability of guardians. Will the stress of taking on additional children cause a breakup or hostility between the couple?

3. Religious and moral convictions. Do you agree with the guardians' philosophies and spiritual and moral views?

4. Financial stability. While the child's inheritance should help with the cost of raising them, it will not last forever. Can the guardians afford to care for your children?

5. Will the guardians also be in charge of the estate? Are the guardians sensible, financially responsible persons, able to handle their own finances, not to mention managing your children's inheritance?

6. Are these the people you would want to adopt your child? Would this be the ideal couple, other than yourselves, to be parents to your child?

Always consult potential guardians before naming them in the will. Give them a chance to consider what it would mean. If it is a friend or friends who you decide on, would they be willing to maintain contact with the child's extended family?

It is an act of loving preparation to write a will for yourselves as a couple and for the security of your child-to-be.

## SUGGESTED READING

*The Parents' Financial Survival Guide*
Theodore E. Hughes and David Klein
Price, Stern and Sloan, 1987

*Sprouse's Income Tax Handbook*
Mary L. Sprouse
Penguin, 1989

*Shopaholics: Serious Help for Addicted Spenders*
Janet Damon
Price, Stern and Sloan, 1988

*How to Stop Fighting About Money and Make Some*
Adriane Berg
Newmarket Press, 1988

*Your Financial Security*
Sylvia Porter
William Morrow and Co. Inc., 1987

*Every Woman's Guide to Profitable Investing*
Elizabeth M. Fowler
AMACOM, 1986

*A Family Guide to Wills, Funerals, and Probate*
Theodore Hughes and David Klein
Scribners, 1983

*Strategy for Personal Finance*
Larry Lang
McGraw-Hill, 1988

## RESOURCE GROUPS

Bankcard Holders of America
460 Spring Park Place
Suite 1000
Herndon, VA 22070
703-481-1100

Council of Better Business Bureaus
4200 Wilson Boulevard
Arlington, VA 22203
202-393-8000

American Financial Services Association
1101 14th Street, N.W.
Dept. DB
Washington, D.C. 20005


"The Student Guide"
Consumer Information Center
Dept. L-10
Pueblo, CO 81009


"Consumer Resource Handbook"
Consumer Information Center
Dept. 578 V
Pueblo, CO 81009


Foundation for Financial Planning
2 Concourse Parkway
Suite 800
Atlanta, GA 30328
404-768-8726


"Wise Home Buying Tips"
U.S. Government Printing Office
710 N. Capital Street
Washington, D.C. 20001


OOPS (Insurance Information Institute)
1-800-221-4954


Health Insurance Association of America
P.O. Box 41455
Washington, D.C. 20018
202-223-7780


"Consumers' Financial Guide"
Securities and Exchange Commission
202-272-7040

U.S. Department of Labor, Pension and Welfare Benefits Department
200 Constitution Avenue
Room N5666
Washington, D.C. 20210
202-523-8921

CHAPTER 12

# OLDER PARENTS

*"With the ancient is wisdom; and in length
of days understanding"*

Job 12:12

## PARENTHOOD AND A FINE WINE: OLDER BUT BETTER?

Some things are better aged, like wine, cheese, and classic cars. But when it comes to people making little people at an advanced age, the pros and cons should be carefully considered.

A woman knows that someday she will no longer be able to conceive. Obstetricians refer to a pregnant woman of 35 years or older as being of "advanced maternal age," or a mature gravida. From 1970 to 1979, the number of women waiting longer before conceiving their first baby almost doubled. The trend to wait has definitely been set. Different factors determine this desire to delay childbearing. Some are careers, finances, fertility or infertility, and late or second marriages.

Does waiting affect the couple once they are ready? It can. Fertility, or the ability to produce a baby, is decreased with a woman's age (see chap. 13). This means that a woman's chance of conceiving, carrying, and delivering a healthy baby decreases with age.

Studies indicate that the older woman choosing to become pregnant may have a higher chance of miscarriage. With an increase in age, there is also an increased likelihood of chromosomal defects, leading to birth defects.

It is also possible that a perfectly normal fetus could be miscarried because of the age of the mother's uterus. For some women, the age of eggs and/or uterus may be enough to cause a miscarriage. This is a great loss for any woman wanting a baby. It is even more tragic for the woman working against her biological clock.

One of the medical problems that may tend to occur more frequently in the older mother is high blood pressure. For example, only 6 percent of 25-year-old first-time mothers may encounter problems with blood pressure during pregnancy. At 35 years of age, the figure increases to 9 percent, and by the time a woman is 40, it is as high as 15 percent. So it is important for the older mother-to-be to be aware of these potential problems.

Having high blood pressure during pregnancy may lead to problems with the placenta. This is the organ that is housed in the uterus and is the filtering system and life source for the baby. If the placenta has defects, it could affect the well-being of the baby. Careful monitoring by a care giver experienced in high-risk pregnancies may help arrest any problems associated with age and blood pressure.

Older mothers tend to have more labor complications. Studies of first-time older mothers show the likelihood of a difficult labor. The explanation, according to one study, is that with the increase in age, the uterine muscle becomes more fiberlike and is not able to contract and relax efficiently. This makes the labor process long and sometimes not too productive. It is understandable, therefore, that the rate of cesarean sections also increases among older mothers.

Any of these factors influencing the ease of pregnancy and childbirth may discourage the older couple from pregnancy. The mature mother-to-be does have special considerations. She must understand that she will need close monitoring by a specialist in high-risk pregnancies. She should seek association with a medical center that is equipped to handle this type of pregnancy.

### Tests for the Older Mother

The older mother-to-be will be asked to consider undergoing special prenatal tests. Probably the most common test is for Down's syndrome, a disorder associated most commonly with older mothers. (See chap. 13 for tests and their implications.)

With any testing comes a risk to the safety of the baby. It also means that the couple must decide what to do if tests show that she is carrying a defective child. If that type of decision-making seems impossible, the couple should reconsider consenting to any testing.

If the tests are done early in the pregnancy, the couple may be asked to decide on a therapeutic abortion. For the older couple, this means the loss of a pregnancy that may have taken months or years to achieve. It may mean having to work even harder to get pregnant again. The pros and cons should be weighed when testing is discussed.

## ADVANTAGE OF AGE

With all the negatives about conceiving at a later age, what is good about being older parents? Many things.

More than likely, the older couple is stable. The woman probably has established a support system and has actually planned the pregnancy. She has her education behind her and a stable career or job. The couple would most likely be economically secure.

The older mother may be more patient and possess sensible judgment. She has probably achieved most of her goals and would be content to try mothering. She has waited for this pregnancy and understands what mothering may involve.

Mature mothers actually may have a positive influence on their child's IQ. The mother's education has been shown to affect the child's intelligence. Infant mortality (death) and Sudden Infant Death Syndrome (SIDS) occur less often to the children of older couples.

The older mother to-be and her partner may feel awkward and wonder why all the fuss about their age. The obstetric health team wants nothing more than to work with the couple in achieving their dream of becoming parents. Early prenatal care, careful monitoring by your care giver, and your desire for a positive outcome are the ingredients needed to help assure you of a healthy pregnancy and baby.

## YOUR PARTNER'S AGE: CAN IT MAKE A DIFFERENCE?

The Bible records that Adam, the first man, was 130 years old at the birth of his third son, Seth. After that, he lived another 807 years and had other sons and daughters. He died at the age of 912. At a time when procreation was the main mission for this first father, it is understandable why he was allowed to live so long and be so fruitful.

Today's men should consider fatherhood at more reasonable ages. But how important is age in the role of being a father? There are pros and cons to being older and receiving the title of "Dear OLD Dad."

Women over 35 are considered potentially high risks for pregnancy. What about the men who are fathers at an older age? Research has been exploring the age factor in sperm quality as well. Just as a woman's eggs age and become unhealthy, so it is believed that a man's undeveloped sperm can also suffer the effects of age. Typically, women stop conceiving between the ages of 40 and 45. This is nature's way of preventing the use of eggs that have been in existence since the woman was born.

What about the man's biological clock? While it has been neither recognized nor acknowledged as existing, it is ticking away just the same.

Researchers now debate whether the age of the father is linked to the production a child with Down's syndrome. Studies in Germany obtained prenatal data involving women 35 years old or older. Researchers stated that the older fathers had an influence on increasing the risk of producing Trisomy 21, or Down's syndrome. One researcher, impressed by the possibility of paternal age influence, advises his patients to have an amniocentesis if the father is over 41. If a woman and her mate are in those high-risk years of over 35, it is difficult to conclude who may be the producer of the extra chromosome leading to Down's syndrome.

A man who is older may decide to marry a younger woman. It may be his second marriage and family and her first. This is now an area of concern for those researchers looking into the paternal age influence.

What does all this research and age difference really mean? That the age of the father may or may not influence the baby's outcome. If the potential father is forty or older, the couple may want to consult a physician with their concerns about paternal age influence.

## COMFORTABLE AT TWO, CROWDED AT THREE

"No man is an island . . . ." And while no couple is an island, there is a fine line between comfortable and crowded when a baby comes along.

Life-style patterns tend to be deeply rooted in the older couple. If longevity of the relationship is a factor, the transition into parenthood may be difficult. As new parents, you are not only making personal adjustments but are taking on a dependent and sometimes noisy roommate.

As you and your partner prepare preconceptionally, discuss those areas of your life that you think will change. Leisure time and flexibility seem to be the areas hardest hit in parenthood. Careers for both parents may feel the strain of nights of interrupted sleep.

Spontaneity and desire in your sex life may be affected temporarily. Generalized role changes must occur, and that takes time. But good news—the older couple tends to adjust well to the late arrival. What may feel like restriction to younger, less experienced couples may very well feel like a welcome change to the older couple. For any couple considering pregnancy, young or old, changes and adjustments should be expected.

## GREAT EXPECTATIONS

Are the expectations of pregnancy and parenthood different for women and their partners who wait to have their first child? As was noted before, feeling like their pregnancy may be the last chance they have may create unrealistic expectations.

The older mother-to-be wants everything to be just perfect. She may feel the need to be the perfect obstetric patient, Lamaze student, and all-natural mother. She reads and exercises and studies prenatal books and pamphlets. Her desire to make it a perfect pregnancy drives her to increase her knowledge and to ask questions.

It is good for you to become educated and responsible for your pregnancy. The information and advice, however, could become overwhelming, almost confusing. It is important to consult your care giver before trying anything you read or hear. An obstetrician trained in high-risk pregnancies will be able to help you assess what advice is safe for you and your baby.

What about parenting? It is probable that the educated, older, and wiser parents will expect great things from their offspring. Once again, the goal may be to make their child a superchild. It may be the older couple's only chance to succeed in parenting. What happens to these children is sometimes devastating. Children become old at a young age and can suffer from stress just like their parents.

We have all heard of musical prodigies who play the violin at age 2. Or how about the preschooler who is pushed into learning elementary subjects like math and science? Mothers are reading articles about educating their child in utero. Promotion of culture and knowledge is a wonderful thing, but children need to be children first.

## LEARNING FROM YOUR CHILD

Perhaps the most endearing charm of a child is his ability to teach his parents how to be children again. Ants on the ground, clouds in the sky, and spring's first flowers become rediscoveries for parents through their children's eyes. The older parents-to-be will want to dust off those old sneakers for the wonderful return to childhood, courtesy of their own children.

## SUGGESTED READING

*The Pregnancy After Thirty Workbook*
Gail Brewer
Rodale Press, 1978

*The Cesarean Birth Experience*
B. Donovan
Beacon Press, 1978

*Silent Knife: Cesarean Prevention and Vaginal Birth after Cesarean*
Nancy Wainer Cohen and Lois Estner
J. F. Bergin, 1983

*Essential Exercises for the Childbearing Year*
Elizabeth Noble
Houghton Mifflin, 1982

## RESOURCE GROUPS

Cesarean Prevention Movement (CPM)
P.O. Box 152
Syracuse, NY 13210
315-424-1942

Cesareans/Support, Education and Concern (C/SEC)
22 Forest Road
Framingham, MA 01701
508-877-8266

CHAPTER 13

# PREPARED FOR THE UNEXPECTED

*"I have learned this at least by my experiment: that if one advances
confidently in the direction of his dreams, and endeavors to live
the life which he has imagined, he will meet with a success
unexpected in common hours."*
—Henry David Thoreau

## WHEN YOU WANT IT AND CAN'T GET IT: PREGNANT

You have made healthy mind, body, and life-style changes, and now you
are ready to get pregnant. We have all known women who talk about
becoming pregnant, and BOOM—they are. For whatever reason, for
some, preconceptional planning goes smoothly, and for others, it is
more of a challenge. Infertility, or difficulty in conceiving, can be both
stressful and disappointing. It is not only a biological problem but a psychological and social problem as well.

Approximately 80 percent of women and their partners attempting to
become pregnant will do so in the first year. Another 9 percent will conceive within the second or third year. Approximately 11 percent have a
problem with infertility. Almost half of all infertility problems involve
the woman, and about one-third of the problems involve the man. A
small percentage involves both partners, which can make it twice as
stressful.

While infertility is a subject that is talked about more and more, a
lack of social support remains. It is still not recognized by society as a
true loss for couples. When couples talk about the future, the possibility
of children is usually present. When the preparations are made and the
time seems right, the dreams of parenthood begin. Looking at baby
clothes, surveying the spare room as a potential nursery, and anticipation of pregnancy and the birth process are all part of the dream that
makes conception so important.

The biological reasons for infertility can be based on a number of
factors:

*Age*: With the peak of fertility occurring between ages 20 and 25, couples waiting until they are in their mid to late thirties may have difficulty conceiving.

*Endometriosis*: More common in women in their thirties, this condition involves the uterine lining migrating into the abdominal cavity. It can cause pain, scarring, and the formation of cysts. As many as 25 to 35 percent of all infertile women suffer from this condition.

*Damaged Reproductive Tracts*: Damage from sexually transmitted diseases, in both men and women, results in difficulty in conceiving.

*Methods of Birth Control*: Devices such as the intrauterine device (IUD) can cause pelvic inflammatory disease. This can cause scarring and adhesions of the reproductive tract. Extended use of birth control pills may make conception more difficult when desired.

*Environmental and Chemical Influences*: Drugs, alcohol, smoking, medications like DES, and exposure to environmental agents like Agent Orange, a defoliant, can all influence the success of conception.

*Physical Health*: Poor nutrition as well as vigorous exercise can influence the ability to conceive.

*Stress*: Stress can inhibit ovulation or even cause the fallopian tubes to clamp down. When that happens, the sperm are unable to reach the egg, which must be fertilized in the tube. Stress can render a man incapable of achieving an erection as well as inhibit the production of mature sperm.

While pregnancy may appear to be an easily achievable state, it is evident that many factors influence how soon or if it occurs. By definition, infertility is one year of unprotected intercourse without conception. After this time, a couple may choose to seek help from the woman's gynecologist or a fertility specialist.

It is important to remain optimistic yet realistic and communicative during this frustrating time. It is important for the woman and her partner to approach their quest for pregnancy together from the onset. Each will individually be tested.

It is important to agree from the beginning that neither is at fault for the difficulty in conceiving. It is a time for the couple to evaluate the strength of their relationship and to decide how far they will go to achieve pregnancy. Testing and fertilization procedures can be quite costly, and they are not always covered by insurance. Time away from work and each other may influence the decision as to how far to take this potentially disappointing quest.

The beginning of the journey toward becoming pregnant should be at the door of a fertility clinic. Such facilities are staffed with doctors, nurses, and therapists who understand the desire of the infertile couple. Seeking a clinic that is close to home and has a good reputation will be the first consideration. The next is to enter the doors and be willing to be comfortable with questions, testing, and frustrations.

## FERTILITY SPECIALISTS: NO SECRETS

It is important not only to like the specialist you plan to work with but to trust her as well. If, for some reason, either of those qualities is missing, look further.

Workups for infertility make take months. The infertility team will need accurate information from the couple as well as their patience. They should be sensitive to the frustrations and concerns of the infertile couple. A complete physical as well as a history of both partners will be necessary.

### History

One of the first tests the infertile couple will encounter is their test of knowledge. Questions will focus on past medical problems well as reproductive health. The following questions probably will be asked.

**For the woman:**
Did you ever have an abortion? Did you ever have abdominal surgery? When? What for?

**For the man:**
Were you ever exposed to Agent Orange, as in Vietnam? Do you take hot baths, or sit for long periods of time?

**For both partners:**
Is there a history of infections of the reproductive tract?
Did your mother take the medication DES when she was pregnant with you? Are you taking any medications? What for? What is the name of the medication?
Do you come in contact with lead, chemicals, radioactive substances, or other hazardous materials where you work or reside?
Do you live in an area sprayed with pesticides?
Do you use a lubricant during intercourse? If so, what is it?

While we may not give much thought to how we make love, this dimension of sexuality is very important. Technique may make the difference if a woman conceives or not. Use of lubricants like K-Y jelly or Surgilube may interfere with the sperm's ability to reach the egg for fertilization. Neither of these two lubricants are contraceptives, and yet both have an effect on the sperm. If there is a need for added lubrication, use vegetable oils or glycerin. Anticipation of some of the questions that may be asked may help the infertile couple to recount their medical history.

## Semen Analysis

Probably the first test performed will be a semen analysis. For this procedure, the man is asked to ejaculate into a container at the physician's office. The semen is checked for its volume, the number of sperm, their shape, and how they move around. It may be necessary for the man to submit two to three samples during the evaluation period.

The characteristics of sperm can be influenced by different factors. Alcohol and smoking have been proven to affect the quality of sperm. If there is a problem with the semen analysis, the man will probably continue to be counseled.

## Postcoital Test

This test is used to determine the receptiveness of the mucous in the cervical area to sperm. Normally at the time of ovulation, the mucous is watery and abundant. This is important for the sperm's ability to swim through the cervix, up the uterus, and out the fallopian tubes. The woman and her partner will be asked to chart when they anticipate ovulation and have intercourse at that time.

The woman must then be checked by the doctor within eight hours after intercourse. The doctor will gather samples of the cervical mucous and put the specimen on a slide. He will view the sample under the microscope.

This test helps determine the amount of mucous produced and its quality. It also determines how many sperm have entered the mucous and if they are alive and moving about.

If the mucous is too thick, the doctor may choose to treat it by giving the woman low doses of estrogen. It is to be taken at specific times during the woman's cycle. The doctor will give instructions as to when to take the medication and any possible side effects.

If the cervix appears to have any problems from past infections or inflammations, the doctor may choose to treat it as well. While poor mucous quality is not an absolute reason for infertility, it can influence the possibility of conception.

Treatment used for thick cervical mucous, or a low sperm count, may include intrauterine insemination (IUI). This procedure involves collecting the semen from the man so that it can be "washed" and concentrated. This is done with special equipment and can be done easily in the doctor's office. The sample is then put into a syringe, which is connected to a thin catheter and inserted through the cervix. The doctor injects the concentrated semen directly into the uterus. This way, the cervical area is avoided altogether, and the sperm have a jump on their long journey toward the fallopian tubes.

## Endometrial Biopsy

This test checks the quality of the endometrium, the lining of the uterus. It is a simple procedure that can be performed at the clinic or in the doctor's office. The doctor inserts an instrument through the cervix and retrieves a small sample of the uterine lining. It is important for the lining to be healthy tissue as it will be the home of the embryo for nine months and supply it with the nourishment it needs to thrive and grow.

If a woman suffers from endometriosis, she may be treated either by medication or by surgery. This problem affects over one-fourth of all infertile women.

## Laparoscopy

This test, usually done in a hospital, can be performed on an outpatient basis. It involves the creation of a small incision near the umbilicus, or belly button. With the woman sedated, the doctor inflates the abdominal cavity with gas. He then inserts a lighted scope into the small opening. He is able to see the uterus, the tubes, and the ovaries. Any scars or adhesions can be visualized and evaluated as possible causes for infertility.

After he evaluates the reproductive organs, he will remove the scope and assist the gas out of the abdominal cavity. He will stitch the small opening, and usually all that is needed is a Band Aid for a dressing.

This test will help the doctor visually evaluate any abnormalities of the outside of the reproductive organs. If the woman has had a history of pelvic inflammatory disease or previous surgery, scarring and adhesions may be present. This may mean the fragile ovaries and fallopian tubes are damaged or altered. This laparoscopic procedure will enable the doctor to make decisions about what the next step toward fertility will be.

## Hysterosalpingogram

This test, which involves injecting dye into the uterus and fallopian tubes, is done in the X-ray department with the aid of fluoroscopy. The doctor can see the shape of the uterus and the patency, or state of being unobstructed, of the tubes. The reproductive organs are highlighted and made more easily visible.

Be sure to ask about this procedure. If you have a history of allergies to dyes, be sure to tell your doctor. The discomfort is minimal. It may be necessary for the doctor to grasp the cervix in order to place the catheter for the injection of the dye.

## Basal Body Temperature

This is one of the few tests a woman can perform on herself without a doctor present. Because pregnancy only occurs at the time a woman ovulates, it is important to know exactly when that is. Basal body temperature, or BBT, charts will help a woman monitor her cycle and the changes she experiences. BBT, usually lower than the normal 98.6° F, is determined by taking either an oral or a rectal temperature before arising in the morning. The activity of getting up and moving about can give altered readings. There are BBT thermometers available commercially.

Ovulation can be determined by several factors:

*Mucous Changes*: The cervical mucous becomes thin and watery and more abundant.

*Mittlesmertz*: This means "midcycle pain," which indicates the ovary's release of an egg. Some women feel a sharp pain on either side of their abdomen.

*Increased Desires*: This is true for many, but not everyone experiences an increase in the need for sex.

*Temperature Changes*: Temperature changes are influenced by hormones released to cause ovulation. It is believed the egg is probably released a day before the first elevation in temperature. The temperature will continue to rise for the next 11 to 16 days, dropping off at the onset of the woman's next period.

Once the woman is able to chart her BBT for perhaps two to three cycles, she will be better able to determine ovulation. Having intercourse three to four days before predicted ovulation and two to three days after may increase the likelihood of pregnancy. It may mean having intercourse for five to seven days in a row.

Charting the BBT is still something you can do at home, and may just work for you. The doctor may advise you to chart your BBT as part of the initial treatment for your infertility. He may also want you to note on what days you have intercourse.

## Hormones

Hormones influence the development and functioning of the reproductive system. One way to determine if the hormones are irregularly functioning is by the menstrual cycle. Women who have irregular periods may need to be assisted with medication. It is not always possible to know if ovulation is occurring in a woman with an irregular cycle.

Menstruation is the indicator that fertilization did not take place. It is not an indicator as to whether ovulation occurred. Medications such as Clomid or Pergonal can be used to start ovulation or increase the frequency of ovulation.

The use of fertility drugs has been shown to increase ovulation within three months. These drugs cannot, however, control how many eggs are released during ovulation. This increases the possibility of conceiving more than one baby. These drugs are also used to prepare a woman for fertilization procedures.

Once the problem is diagnosed, it is then up to the couple to decide what to do. The doctor should be able to tell you what treatment is available for your infertility problem. You should also find out the success rates of the treatments he prescribes, as well as the cost and time it will consume.

It is difficult at this time to have to consider money. If, however, the treatment's chances for success are small, and the treatment is very expensive, how far do you pursue your dream? It is difficult to be practical at a time when your emotions seem to rule.

You and your partner will need to discuss your options and agree upon a decision. Make the right choice for you with the knowledge your physician can offer.

## VARIATIONS ON CONCEPTION

There are a number of ways to conceive a baby in these days of medical miracles.

## In Vitro Fertilization (IVF)

IVF is the creation of a fertilized egg outside the mother's body. The woman may be given fertility drugs to increase her ovulation frequency and the number of eggs her ovary releases. The doctor performs a laparoscopic examination at the time of ovulation. He will harvest, or gather, the eggs off the surface of the ovary. He places them in a petri dish, a special container with a substance that aids in the growth of life.

He then places the father's sperm in the dish with the eggs. After the egg or eggs are fertilized, the doctor places a thin tube through the cervical opening and injects the fertilized egg into the uterus. The egg, now an embryo, then finds a place to implant itself and begins to grow.

A few drawbacks to IVF include:

- A success rate of 13 percent.
- The cost is not covered by insurance.
- The medications the woman must take may cause unpleasant side effects.
- The travel time and work loss of going to the clinic for the procedure.
- The increased chance of a multiple pregnancy.

## Gamete Intrafallopian Transfer (GIFT)

This procedure is similar to IVF. The eggs are harvested from the ovary and mixed with the father's sperm immediately. The actual fertilization of the egg and cell division occur within the woman's body. The eggs and sperm are inserted into the woman's fallopian tubes, where the fertilization must take place. After fertilization, the egg then drifts down into the uterus and implants itself in the uterine lining.

The success rates vary from 27 to 40 percent. The natural occurrence of fertilization and cell division in the body seems to be a selling point for couples.

## Artificial Insemination

This procedure can be performed with either the partner's semen or that of anonymous donor.

### *Artificial Insemination by Husband (AIH)*

Artificial insemination by husband requires real teamwork. The woman must be ovulating and her partner must produce semen on command. The semen is introduced into the uterus by a thin catheter that is inserted by the doctor through the cervix.

This direct deposit of sperm into the uterus increases the number of sperm getting to the egg, which is waiting in the tube. The couple must remain in open communication and attempt to relax, and yes, find humor wherever they can.

### Artificial Insemination by Donor (AID)

Artificial insemination by donor is an alternative available if the man's sperm count is too low for conception by AIH or he has a genetic disease that he does not want to pass on. AID presents new concerns to the infertile couple. They will have to decide whether to tell the child how he was conceived. The anonymity of the donor will not allow the child to pursue his "biological" father. These concerns should be thought out by the couple considering AID.

How does the partner feel about his mate carrying another man's child? Sounds like a silly question when you have both wanted a baby so badly. Nonetheless, it is better to consider all the concerns before undergoing the insemination.

Although the donors are screened, they may not have told the whole truth about their medical history. As with the blood donor scare concerning AIDS, fears of the unknown may trouble the couple considering artificial insemination. On the positive side, there is a 50 to 80 percent success rate over a one-year period with artificial insemination.

Once all the concerns and questions are answered, the couple should come to an agreement on which means of fertilization is right for them.

## Surrogate Mothering

When fertilization or pregnancy is impossible for the woman but the man is fertile, some couples have decided on surrogate mothering. This avenue for becoming parents is nontraditional and can be complicated.

The couple should first decide whom they would like to carry their child. Some couples prefer someone they know. Many times, family members and friends are more than willing to consider being a surrogate. The couple and prospective surrogate must examine some difficult questions.

First, the prospective mother should be sure she will not feel awkward about carrying the child of her sister's or best friend's husband. Another difficulty with family or friend surrogates may be the amount of contact after the baby is born. If the surrogate is married with children of her own, it may be difficult for her family to adjust.

There are advantages in knowing who will carry the baby. Knowledge of the background, health history, and maturity of the mother gives an added security. However, the surrogate's psychological well-being, whether she is a friend, family member, or an anonymous surrogate, must be assessed carefully.

There are court battles between surrogates and the biological father and his infertile wife. Perhaps the most widely publicized case is that of Baby "M." While the decision of who is right and who is wrong lies with the courts, the issue is clearly a difficult one. Because the woman is basically giving up her baby for adoption, she can change her mind at the last moment. This is probably the greatest concern of the couple considering surrogate mothering.

An anonymous surrogate can be chosen through an agency that finds surrogates for infertile couples. These agencies can be expensive. The couple should be prepared to ask many questions. Some of these are:

- Will there be contact between the surrogate and the couple during the pregnancy?
- How much will the surrogate and agency be paid? Will that include all expenses, prenatal visits, and paperwork?
- What are the legal rights of the couple and the surrogate throughout the pregnancy and after the birth? Do you need a lawyer?
- What type of health and psychological counseling are performed on the surrogate?
- What type of counseling is available for the infertile couple?
- What type of emotional support will the surrogate receive after the baby is born?

The difficulties in surrogate mothering must be weighed carefully against the advantages. The child will be genetically connected to the father. The infertile mother must be prepared for the fact that this child, however strongly desired, is still biologically not her child.

It is then necessary for the infertile mother to file for adoption of the child. The couple will have to decide if or when they disclose to their child her means of conception. While this issue can be dealt with at a later date, it is still a consideration preconceptionally.

The complications of surrogacy are probably most serious in the legal sense. While couples may think that a child is all they really want, they should consider the unexpected outcomes.

A case in Michigan demonstrates the tragedy of surrogacy. A

woman, having agreed to become a surrogate, was to be paid $10,000 on the birth of the child. Her child was born with a birth defect, possibly indicating mental retardation. The child needed additional treatment for an infection it acquired in the hospital. The biological father wanted treatment withheld. The surrogate mother had no maternal feelings for the child. The hospital received a court order and did treat the baby.

A few weeks later, the paternity of the child was checked by blood testing. It was proven that the woman's husband fathered the child. Apparently she was unaware of her pregnancy at the time of insemination. The woman kept the baby, and the infertile couple withheld the money. To add insult to injury, the couple has a lawsuit pending against the surrogate mother for millions of dollars.

In all of the controversy surrounding surrogacy, it would appear that the child's best interest may not be at the top of the list. Couples must be stable and knowledgeable before pursuing surrogacy. State laws vary and need careful investigation to protect all those involved, especially the child.

## NOTHING IS PERFECT

Technology has been the link between infertile couples and parenthood. While the road may be long and emotionally draining for the infertile couple, it may not be free of further disappointments.

For anyone considering pregnancy, the desire for a healthy baby is probably top priority. The truth is that once fertilization occurs, there is still no guarantee of a "normal" baby. There are several known factors that influence the health of a baby.

The mother's health is probably the most obvious influence on a baby's health. As was discussed earlier, it is important for the preconceptional woman to have a clean bill of health before she conceives. If she has a history of a medical condition, she should be sure to consult her physician before becoming pregnant. The woman's age is also an influencing factor.

Each child conceived is an equal combination of his mother's and father's chromosomes. If, for some reason, there is a defective gene in the chromosome, a child may be born with either physical or psychological disabilities. For anyone with the potential of producing a genetically defective child, genetic counseling may be an option.

Genetic counseling will provide the high-risk couple with information and support. The couple can learn what tests are available to diagnose genetically linked problems. A woman's obstetrician should be able to recommend a counselor in this field.

Below are some of the more common genetically related disorders.

*Down's Syndrome (Trisomy 21).* This disorder involves a defect of the twenty-first chromosome, which leads to characteristics of physical malformations and some degree of mental retardation. There is a high incidence in older mothers. It is not treatable.

*Huntington's Chorea.* This is a hereditary disease of the brain, characterized by jerky movements, speech disturbances, and mental deterioration. It usually appears between the ages of thirty and forty-five. Deterioration occurs over a period of time, leading to incapacitation and death.

*Cystic Fibrosis.* A hereditary disease characterized by the accumulations of thick mucous in the lungs and abnormal secretions of sweat. It is a recessive trait, meaning both parents must possess the gene in order for the disease to manifest.

It is treatable but not curable. Life expectancy is in the twenties. A sweat test is used to diagnose CF.

*Spina Bifida.* This disorder has a 5 percent incidence related to a familial history. The spinal column does not fuse during fetal development, allowing the cord to protrude through the opening.

Also known as a neural tube defect, spina bifida can be detected prenatally by testing. The extent of bulge of the cord through the spinal column opening determines how difficult it would be to repair the defect. The ability to use the lower limbs is also influenced by the severity of the defect. Approximately 60 percent of all cases are operable.

*Hemophilia.* This sex-linked recessive trait is most often transmitted from mother to son. The children bruise easily and have difficulty with clotting of their blood. They must be treated with medication to increase clotting and receive blood transfusions as needed.

Some genetically related defects are specific to ethnic groups. Following are a few of these.

*Tay Sachs.* This disease occurs most frequently among Jewish people originating in Eastern Europe. It is a recessive gene that causes the brain of the child to become firm at about six months of age. The disease causes deterioration of the muscles, seizures, blindness, and other neurological problems that ultimately result in death.

There is a blood test to detect if the parents are carriers. This can be done before conception with amniocentesis. There is no treatment available for Tay Sachs.

*Sickle Cell.* Occurring in about 1 out of 500 blacks in this country, sickle cell is a genetically linked disorder. When oxygen is reduced in the blood stream, the red blood cells change shape, resembling that of a sickle. This causes clumping, which in turn blocks the tiny vessels in the body. This causes severe pain in the area of the blockage. Symptoms can begin as young as two to three months of age. Treatment includes controlling symptoms.

## TESTS FOR GENETIC DEFECTS

With the increase in information available through research, doctors can perform tests preconceptionally, prenatally, and on the newborn. The genetic or chromosomal defect the doctor is looking for will determine when he will perform testing and which test he will use.

Some tests are as simple as blood work, while some can be quite complicated. It is important to understand what they involve and the risks, as the tests are used to diagnose problems, not necessarily correct them. The couple should understand that they may even be asked to decide on keeping or aborting the fetus, should it be found abnormal.

### Amniocentesis

This test is performed during pregnancy. Amniotic fluid is extracted from the uterus with a long, thin needle. Ultrasound is used during the test to visualize where the placenta and baby are located.

This test is usually performed after the thirteenth week of pregnancy, with results available at weeks nineteen or twenty. Such disorders as Down's syndrome, spina bifida, and cystic fibrosis can be detected.

### Chorionic Villi Sampling (CVS)

This relatively new procedure extracts cells from the growing placenta by using a needle inserted into the abdomen of the mother. The advantage is that it can be performed early in the pregnancy, with results available between weeks six and eleven. That way if a defect is found, an abortion can be performed.

Disorders that can be diagnosed by CVS are the same as diagnosed by an amniocentesis.

## Ultrasonography

This procedure is pain-free and performed in the radiology department of a hospital. Sound waves bounced off the uterine contents create an image on a screen. Skeletal defects and other major structural defects can be diagnosed.

This test is often used to determine the gestational age of the fetus. There are no risks associated with this test.

## Alpha Fetoprotein Screening (AFP)

This blood test is to detect neural tube defects like spina bifida and chromosomal abnormalities. Protein produced by the baby's liver is found in the mother's blood. There are high levels of AFP in women carrying a child with certain birth defects. The AFP is lower than normal in other disorders including Down's syndrome. The test is done between weeks fifteen and twenty.

## Percutaneous Umbilical Blood Sampling (PUBS)

This test is used during late pregnancy and gives indications of the same disorders found through amniocentesis and CVS. The difference is that blood is withdrawn from the umbilical vein. A sample is obtained by inserting a needle into the mother's abdomen and then into the umbilical cord.

Doctors can diagnose and perform some treatments on the baby in utero. Blood transfusions or needed medications can be given to the baby to treat problems diagnosed through PUBS.

These tests are wonderful advancements in prenatal technology. They do, however, invariably leave the couple to decide the fate of their unborn child. It is important to discuss the nature of the test, its risks, and what the results mean.

The decision to terminate the pregnancy, especially if it was not easily obtained, could be an emotionally charged situation. The woman and her partner should carefully consider this option and agree without doubt that it is or is not the best choice for them.

Occasionally, these tests can predict abnormalities that can be treated in utero. Under specially trained professionals, corrective procedures have been performed, and babies have been spared. Blood transfusions have been given to fetuses, as well as other minor corrective surgery. Technological advances will in time be able to give hope to more couples carrying a defective child.

# MISCARRIAGE

The medical term is spontaneous abortion. The emotional term is loss of a dream. Approximately 15 to 20 percent of all pregnancies end in miscarriage. Below are a few factors believed to contribute to the incidence of miscarriage.

## Age

Chances of miscarriage increase with the increased age of the mother. At age 25, there is a 15 percent chance; while at age 40, there is a 31 percent chance.

## Occupation

While most jobs present little threat to a pregnancy, some industries expose employees to hazardous substances. Fumes, solvents, some metals, and chemicals are all possible causes for spontaneous abortions.

## Health

Poor health habits including poor nutrition, smoking, alcohol consumption, taking medications, or a preexisting medical condition may increase the likelihood of a pregnancy loss.

Research has been able to disprove beliefs about other factors as causes of miscarriages. Some of those include use of the pill or IUD, a previous elective abortion, sexual intercourse, and active exercising.

A miscarriage is a sign that the developing baby had something wrong with it, such as a genetic imperfection. Early abortions occur between the seventh and fourteenth weeks. Late abortions occur between weeks seventeen and twenty-eight. Usually in these cases, it is a problem with the placenta, uterus, or a cervix that opened too soon.

However it may be explained, it is still a devastating loss to the couple. The woman is experiencing physical as well as emotional pain. The man, too, experiences emotional pain, which may be expressed as anger or resentment. The couple may be overwhelmed by the medical aspects of the miscarriage. It is important for them to ask questions and seek help in understanding this loss.

It is natural and healthy to treat a miscarriage as a loss and mourn. Whether the pregnancy was planned or not, grief is to be expected; it is part of the healing process. Some couples choose to hold a special service with friends and family.

Our society does not provide support to couples suffering from a miscarriage. Rituals such as funerals or wakes are observed for the dead. But the loss of a child, whether it is only a few weeks in gestational age or a baby born without life, is a loss of someone loved.

If there is any comfort to be found, it is in the fact that a miscarriage does not affect the chances for another pregnancy. Studies show that because the woman's body has the ability to recognize imperfection in a fetus, most likely her next baby will be normal.

As with any crisis, feelings between the couple should be shared openly and honestly. For the infertile couple who have finally achieved pregnancy, this loss may seem unbearable. Unless otherwise advised, the couple should not give up their dream of becoming parents.

## ECTOPIC PREGNANCY

An ectopic, or tubal, pregnancy is both physically and emotionally painful. Like a miscarriage, it possesses many emotional aspects, sometimes difficult to handle.

A tubal pregnancy occurs when the fertilized egg implants in the fallopian tube instead of descending into the uterus. It begins to grow and eventually ruptures the tube. The woman feels pain and other symptoms that may lead her doctor to decide to remove the ruptured tube through surgery. This, of course, means the woman then has only one tube. This can be very disheartening to the couple who have now had their chance of parenthood decreased by half.

A few reasons that ectopics occur include scar formation or adhesions of the reproductive tract. If a woman has had a history of pelvic inflammatory disease, or any previous abdominal surgery, she may be prone to develop an ectopic pregnancy.

Typically, the symptoms of vaginal bleeding, lower abdominal pain, weakness, and fainting may occur between weeks eight and twelve. If the woman is unaware that she is pregnant, these symptoms may be very confusing to both her and her doctor.

There are several tests the doctor can perform to diagnose an ectopic pregnancy. They include blood work, using a lighted scope (laparoscope) to look into the abdominal cavity, a surgical procedure, ultrasound, or withdrawing fluid from the area surrounding the uterus by using a large thin needle.

Once the condition is diagnosed, the physician will probably act quickly to perform surgery. There is considerable blood loss from a ruptured tube. The tube may or may not be salvageable. If not, it will be removed. The woman may spend four to six days in the hospital.

With the medical crisis over, the couple will experience many feelings of loss. Grief of the loss of the potential child, as well as part of their fertility, is experienced. Anger over the loss of control they feel can lead to difficulties for couples. It is vital for them to be open and honest. This is a frightening experience, and couples should understand that their fears, anger, sorrow, and frustrations are normal.

## OTHER FLOWERS WAITING TO BLOOM

A small percentage of couples will remain infertile. Their feelings about never becoming biological parents can be overwhelming. These couples should seek counseling during this stressful time of their life. To remain strong as a couple, they will need to communicate with each other and work through their feelings together. These couples have one more option remaining.

### Adoption

A lot of emotional pain and energy go into infertility testing and futile attempts at pregnancy. Some couples lose sight of their initial goal of becoming parents. If parenthood is the ultimate goal, the infertile couple must let go of their infertility. They should consider redirecting their energy into exploring the adoption option.

There are several ways a couple can pursue adoption. Independent, agency, and international adoption are the most typical ways.

Independent adoptions are currently legal in forty-four states. The couple makes arrangements with the birth mother through a doctor or lawyer and agrees to pay medical costs of the mother and any legal fees. These adoptions are not meant to be money-making arrangements.

The couple should decide how much contact they want with the birth mother. A complete medical history of the baby's parents and extended family should be acquired. Once in the custody of the adoptive parents, the baby should also be examined thoroughly by a pediatrician.

Agencies act as the go-between for the birth mother and the adoptive parents. They also act as advocates for the child by requiring home studies. These may seem investigative when in reality they are a way for the couple and agency to evaluate the home situation. Agencies want to determine the strength of the marriage, the stability of the home, and the motivation of the parents.

Most couples would probably like to have the Gerber baby placed in their arms, but some couples prefer and accept the challenge of children with special needs. These kids, who are more readily available, include physically or emotionally handicapped children, mentally retarded children, sibling groups, or older children. These children need a strong foundation on which to build their lives.

There are agencies across the United States which deal in international adoptions of children from South Korea, India, Colombia, El Salvador, and Peru. There have been many successful placements through these agencies.

The paperwork and the cost are probably the two primary drawbacks. The cost of $6,000 to $10,000 can be too much for a middle-income couple. The couple may need to travel to the country to pick up the child. Time away from work and expenses add to the cost. Working with an experienced agency is vital for a smooth adoption.

Adoption is an option for infertile couples and yet is not without its concerns. It is not uncommon for adopted children to seek their biological parents when they are older. This may feel threatening to the adoptive parents and should be talked through before considering adoption.

Sometimes extended family members may not be totally supportive, especially in international adoptions. They need time to work through their racial biases and concerns. All of these concerns of adoption should be carefully and openly discussed.

But adoption is still a way for a couple to become a family. In fact, infertile couples can relate better to their adopted child at the time in his life when he becomes aware he is adopted. A child may feel a loss of his biological mother and father and need extra emotional support. The infertile couple knows of loss as well and will be able to help their child through this difficult time. It is almost as if infertile couples and their adopted children were always meant to be together. For it is clear that biology does not create parents; love and desire do.

## SUGGESTED READING

*You Can Have a Baby*
J. H. Bellina and J. Wilson
Crown Publishers, 1985

*The Infertility Book: A Comprehensive Medical and Emotional Guide*
C. Harkness
Volcano Press, 1987

*Understanding: A Guide to Impaired Fertility for Family and Friends*
R. B. Hunt
Perspective Press, 1983

*Miracle Babies and Other Happy Endings*
M. Perloe and L. G. Christie
Rawson Associates, 1986

*New Conceptions: A Consumer's Guide to the Newest Infertility Treatments*
L. B. Andrews
St. Martin's Press, 1984

*In Pursuit of Pregnancy*
J. Liebmann-Smith
Newmarket Press, 1987

*Childless Is Not Less*
V. Love
Bethany House, 1984

*The Penguin Adoption Handbook*
E. B. Bolles
Viking Penguin, 1984

*Adoption: Parenthood Without Pregnancy*
C. Canape
Holt, Rinehart & Winston, 1986

*The Adoption Resource Book*
 L. Gilman
Harper & Row, 1984

*Understanding Artificial Insemination: A Guide for Patients*
W. Schlaff and C. F. Vercollone
RESOLVE, Inc., 1987

*Childless by Choice: Choosing Childlessness in the Eighties*
M. Faux
Doubleday, 1984

*Overcoming Endometriosis*
M. L. Ballweg
Congdon & Weed, 1987

*Coping with Genetic Disorders: A Guide for Counseling*
J. C. Fletcher
Harper & Row, 1982

*The Fertility Question*
M. Nofziger
The Book Publishing Company, 1982

*Making Babies: The New Science and Ethics of Conception*
P. Singer and D. Wells
Scribners, 1985

*Beyond Heartache*
M. Hanes
Tyndale House, 1984

*The Courage to Grieve*
J. Tatelbaum
Harper & Row, 1980

## RESOURCE GROUPS

American Fertility Society
2131 Magnolia Avenue
Suite 201
Birmingham, AL 35256
205-933-8494

Compassionate Friends
P.O. Box 1347
Oak Brook, IL 60521
312-323-5010

DES Action
2845 24th Street
San Francisco, CA 94110
415-826-5060

North American Council on Adoptable Children
810 18th Street, N.W.
Suite 703
Washington, D.C. 20006
202-466-7570

OURS, Inc.
3307 Highway 100 North
Suite 203
Minneapolis, MN 55442
612-535-4829

Parents for Private Adoption
P.O. Box 7
Pawlet, VT 05761

Pregnancy and Infant Loss Center
1415 E. Wayzata Boulevard
Suite 22
Wayzata, MN 55391
612-473-9372

RESOLVE, Inc.
5 Water Street
Arlington, MA 02174
617-643-2424

# CHAPTER 14

# HOOKED ON BIRTH CONTROL

*"No woman can call herself free who does not own and control
her body. No woman can call herself free until she can choose
consciously whether she will or will not be a mother."*
—Margaret Sanger

## SO SAFE SO FAR

We talk, we laugh, we play, and we love. We communicate through
many languages, including our sexuality. Women and men are by nature
sexual beings. Intercourse is just a small part of our sexuality. It is a tool
to create, strengthen, celebrate, and commit ourselves to a relationship.
Our enjoyment of our sexuality is what makes us different from other
living creatures. There is beauty in this wonder and heartache if an
unwanted pregnancy occurs.

Choosing a form of birth control should be the choice and responsibility of the couple. Men and women should be willing to work together
to use the form they choose. The expense of birth control also should be
shared by the couple. Perhaps most important, both the man and the
woman should watch for any side effects from their choice in birth control. While few birth control methods are directly used by the man, he
should be equally involved in the proper use of these techniques.

Knowledge of what is available, how it works, and how it fits in the
couple's life are the first steps in effective birth control. With more than
half of all pregnancies in the United States being unplanned, self-
education along with professional advice is necessary.

Only you know what will work in your life. Your physician can help
you decide if you are a good candidate for such contraceptives as birth
control pills and the IUD. With all that is available, we as a sexual society are still in need of more. Physicians and researchers are seeking
longer lasting and more effective techniques.

### Birth Control Pills

These pills contain hormones that make the body think it is pregnant.

Side effects include nausea, vomiting, breast tenderness, weight gain, and a decreased libido. Women who are over thirty-five and smokers are advised to consider other techniques of birth control. Average cost is from $8.50 to $19.95 per pack.

Pills must be taken every day, and if a day is missed, other means of birth control must be used. They are obtained through a doctor, who must prescribe them. It is necessary to be checked every six months for any cervical changes or problems.

While it is the most effective and popular birth control method, it does not protect from sexually transmitted diseases including AIDS. New, lower doses are making the pill more tolerable to more women.

## Barrier Methods

This group includes condoms, diaphragms, vaginal sponges, and cervical caps. All are designed to keep sperm from reaching the egg.

Condoms should be placed on the erect penis before it touches the vaginal opening. Preejaculatory secretions can be home to millions of sperm. Once ejaculation has taken place, it is important that the man hold the base of the condom as he withdraws from the vagina. This helps prevent any leakage while he is exiting. Condoms have been instrumental in decreasing the incidence of sexually transmitted diseases, including AIDS. Both women and men should carry condoms. They have an average yearly cost of about $30. This, of course, varies according to how often there is intercourse.

A diaphragm is a device that the woman uses. It is a little dome made of latex which she inserts into the vagina and carefully places over the cervix. It requires a doctor to fit a woman for it, as everyone is different in size. It is used in conjunction with a spermicidal jelly. The jelly is placed inside the dome before insertion. After each ejaculation, fresh spermicidal jelly is then inserted with an applicator. It is not necessary to remove the diaphragm immediately, and it is advisable to leave it in for a couple of hours after intercourse.

Vaginal sponges can be purchased in the drugstore in boxes of three or six. The sponge, like the diaphragm, is inserted into the vagina and acts to cover the cervix. It is impregnated with spermicide that is activated by moistening the sponge before inserting it. The sponge has a small string to assist in removal.

A cervical cap is a plasticlike cap that is about one inch in diameter and conforms to the woman's cervix. They are custom fit and made in the doctor's office.

## Intrauterine Device (IUD)

These devices have undergone considerable improvement over the past few years. The IUD is inserted through the cervix into the uterus. It is a foreign object in the uterus which discourages the fertilized egg from implanting in the uterine lining. Treated with hormones, these devices can remain in place for years. A string attached to the device allows the woman to check its placement. The IUD is inserted by a doctor in the office.

Disadvantages of the IUD include the fact that the string acts as a pathway for bacteria to enter the uterus directly. Some women experience an increase in menstrual flow and cramps. In some cases, the IUD may perforate the uterus. There is a 5 percent risk of pregnancy. The IUD does not interfere with foreplay or require daily consideration. It is important to check for the presence of the string routinely, to make sure the IUD does not ascend farther into the uterus or come out.

## Spermicides

A spermicide, a chemical substance that kills sperm, can be in the form of a jelly, foam, or cream. Spermicides should be used in conjunction with a diaphragm, a condom, or even a sponge. They can be used alone but do not have a great success rate for pregnancy prevention. They do not have long-term effects and can be bought in the drugstore. They have an annual price tag of about $50.

Spermicides should be used before each entry of the penis into the vagina. There is an 18 percent risk of pregnancy with this method of birth control.

## Coitus Interruptus (Withdrawal)

This technique requires great willpower on the part of the man. It is his responsibility to withdraw his penis preceding his urge to ejaculate. As was noted before, there are sperm present in the preejaculatory semen, so that withdrawal may not always be foolproof.

This technique focuses on timing, rather than pleasure, in sex. This is not the most reliable means of birth control; the risk of pregnancy and sexually transmitted diseases is high. If this is the means a couple chooses, the man should wash his penis after each ejaculation so as to not introduce any living sperm into the vagina on his next entry.

## Abstinence

As long as both partners agree on it, this technique for birth control is obviously effective. Neither partner should lose sight of the bond that sexual intimacy brings to a relationship. If abstinence is the choice temporarily, then other means of sexual satisfaction should be explored. Mutual masturbation, touching, caressing, holding, and verbal reassurance are necessary.

## Morning-After Pill

Unprotected intercourse during midcycle has 1 to 17 percent chance of resulting in pregnancy. On occasion, when no protection is used, it is possible through a doctor to receive postcoital pills. These pills contain hormones that, when taken within twelve to twenty-four hours after intercourse, will decrease the chance of pregnancy and increase the likelihood of the woman getting her period. This afterthought technique should not be used as a responsible means of birth control. It is exclusively for unprotected, unexpected intercourse.

## Abortion

Abortion is a means to ending an unwanted pregnancy. It is not truly a birth control method and, like postcoital pills, should be used only when absolutely necessary. Sexually active women have a responsibility to themselves to find a birth control method that will prevent them from having to seek an abortion for an unwanted pregnancy.

## Sterilization

The most permanent means of birth control, sterilization can be performed on either the man or the woman. Vasectomy is a procedure that severs the tubes that carry the sperm. A simple procedure, it can be performed in a doctor's office, with minimal discomfort. Before considering vasectomy as an option, the man should understand that reversing this procedure has not been highly successful.

Tubal ligation is the counterpart of the vasectomy. This procedure can be done on an outpatient basis in the operating room. The doctor makes a small incision at the belly button and inserts a laparoscopic instrument for visualization. He can then cut each fallopian tube and remove part of the tube. The incision is closed and a bandage is applied.

This procedure should also be carefully thought through before consent is given. Reversal of such procedures has not had a high success rate and is quite costly.

It must be remembered that vasectomy and tubal ligation are both meant to be permanent means of birth control.

## Natural Family Planning

The advantage of natural family planning is the total control of one's own birth control. It does require a finely tuned awareness of the woman to her body. Our bodies give us signals when changes are occurring. Tuning into the subtle changes will allow the couple to avoid fertile times through abstinence or use of another contraceptive device.

### Basal Body Temperature

This technique requires charting a daily record of the woman's temperature for three to four months. Before arising in the morning, she should lie quietly, take her temperature, and record it.

The BBT drops slightly before ovulation. There is a noticeable temperature increase twenty-four to seventy-two hours after ovulation. By charting for several months, she sees a pattern of when ovulation occurs. It is at this time that intercourse should be avoided. Because sperm can live for two to three days, plenty of time should be allotted before ovulation and after to use other means of contraception.

For example, if Sue had intercourse on Monday and ovulates on Wednesday, it may be possible for her to get pregnant. The sperm may be in the fallopian tubes just waiting for the arrival of the egg. It only takes one sperm to fertilize an egg. For Sue, it may be more realistic to abstain from Monday to Friday, just to be sure.

### Calendar Method

This method requires keeping a menstrual calendar. By documenting each month for six to eight months, a woman can learn what cycle her body is on. Recording the days she menstruates and possibly ovulates will assist her in avoiding fertile times.

A few factors to keep in mind:
- Ovulation occurs 14+ -2 days before the scheduled onset of the next period.
- The sperm can survive for two to three days in the woman's reproductive tract.

- The egg can live for 24 hours.
- The woman should always play safe by using other means if she is not sure of her cycle. Awareness of the reproductive cycle will not only prevent pregnancy but help it to occur when the time is right.

### Mucous Method

The body has a wonderful technique to aid in conception. The cervix, the doorway into the uterus, secretes more mucous during ovulation. Before and after ovulation, women tend to have a more yellowish discharge that also tends to be thick. During ovulation, the discharge becomes clear and slippery, like raw egg white.

Other symptoms of ovulation include a slight pain on either side of the lower abdomen. This is called mittlesmertz, or midcycle pain. This indicates that the egg has ruptured out of the ovary and is being processed into the fallopian tubes, to await fertilization. Some women feel abdominal heaviness and even some rectal discomfort. By tuning into these changes, a woman can avoid intercourse during this time in her cycle.

### Sympto-Thermal Method

Probably the best method is to combine both the symptoms of ovulation and the basal body temperature. The combination of these and careful charting will give added protection to prevent conception.

## THE FUTURE OF BIRTH CONTROL

It is estimated that seventy women out of one thousand receive abortions worldwide per year. The birth control methods available obviously are not meeting the needs of women. With the future of birth control looking so positive, it is hoped that in time abortions will not be such a needed procedure.

The following are some of the goals of birth control:

- It is hoped that with refinement, antifertility products will be available for men, who are equally responsible for conception and the prevention of pregnancy.
- The pill is currently at a low dose, but with time it will be more coordinated with a woman's cycle, possessing fewer side effects as well.
- IUDs will be smaller and more effective. The ability to leave it in place for as long as five to ten years would decrease the risks from removal and reinsertion.

- Sponges, cervical caps, and diaphragms are widely accepted by women. A disposable diaphragm is being studied.
- Long-acting steroid injections to prevent pregnancy are being examined. Protection can last for one, three, or six months.
- Ovulation detection techniques are being studied to allow a woman to predict and protect during her cycle.
- Steroid implants that last up to five years are being experimented with in several countries with a high success rate.
- Vaginal rings with low doses of hormones are being researched and studied. These rings can be left in place for six months or more at a time.
- A pill to inhibit ovulation is in the works. A nasal spray to inhibit fertility in men is being studied as well.

## THE CONS OF CONTRACEPTIVES

For the future of family planning, some of the long-term effects of birth control should be considered. With any means of birth control, except condoms, sexually transmitted diseases can still be spread. With the wide acceptance and use of the pill, the rate of sexually transmitted diseases has increased considerably.

The pill itself has benefited millions of women. It has a high rate of effectiveness but is not without side effects. Perhaps it is not the pill so much as the combination of a woman's health, life-style, and the pill. There are some symptoms to be aware of when using the pill. These include shortness of breath, chest pain, severe headache, abdominal pain, and swelling of the legs.

Women with certain health problems should not use the pill. These include women with a history of poor circulation, liver diseases, liver tumors, abnormal bleeding of the genital area, and cancer of the breast or reproductive tract.

Other women who should avoid the pill are those with high blood pressure, diabetes, sickle cell anemia, renal disease, women over forty, anyone considering elective surgery in the near future, and women who smoke. Women who suffer from depression are advised to consider another form of birth control.

Because the hormones in the pill are synthetic, they may tend to cause various reactions in different organs and systems. On purchasing birth control pills, the woman should read the insert that is required by the Food and Drug Administration to be in each pack of pills. It lists the side effects and advises women to seek medical attention if they suffer from any problems. With continued research on the pill, it is hoped that more women will be able to use it safely and effectively.

The IUD does not involve the use of synthetic hormones, which appeals to women who cannot tolerate these chemicals. These devices were and are still not without side effects. The string that is connected to the IUD and is ever present in the vagina can act as a wide open road for bacteria to travel. The bacteria can be from sexually transmitted diseases or those germs that are not meant to be in the uterus. Infections can cause scarring and the formation of adhesions.

In fact, the way the IUD works is through the uterus's constant battle against the device. It actually creates a chronic inflammation, which allows the white blood cells to accumulate and destroy sperm or the fertilized egg. It creates an environment considered hostile to the fertilized egg, so that implantation does not take place.

Signs that should be reported to your doctor include abdominal pain, increase in temperature, spotting (bleeding between periods), heavy periods, a foul discharge from the vagina, or clots. These signs could mean a serious infection or perforation of the uterus.

Women with a history of reproductive organ problems, blood or coagulation problems, a current pelvic inflammatory disease, or severe menstrual cramps should avoid using an IUD.

It is possible to become pregnant with an IUD in place, which can lead to infection of the uterus and the fetus and usually a miscarriage. This is typically diagnosed during the second trimester (months four through six). If you think you are pregnant, contact your care giver immediately so the IUD can be removed.

If the string cannot be located in the vagina, the IUD may have come out or gone farther into the uterus. The doctor will locate it through manual examination, ultrasound, laparoscope, or perhaps surgery. It is important to check periodically to see that the string is in place.

Sterilization, whether performed on the man or the woman, is foolproof if done correctly. It is the most permanent of birth control methods. Reconstructive surgery for tubal ligations and vasectomies is available, but it is not always successful and can cost thousands of dollars.

Fortunately, researchers are attempting to create a method by which they can plug the fallopian tubes so that fertilization cannot occur. The plugs can be removed when the woman chooses to become pregnant. Until this type of birth control is available, women and men should think carefully before undergoing sterilization. Both partners should be in total agreement, having discussed this procedure in detail before deciding. It should be considered a permanent means of birth control.

## READJUSTMENT UNTIL READY
Let us say that until now you have chosen a birth control just right for you as a couple. You both like it and are responsible for it in one way or another. You have made the choices and changes in your life through preconceptional planning. You have chosen to conceive, and yet when is a safe time, if you have been using a birth control method like the pill or an IUD? Both of these techniques require time off for the body before conception occurs.

The pill, as was noted before, is a synthetic hormone. It has an effect on many of the body's systems. To stop taking the pill one month and expect pregnancy the next may be unreasonable. In fact, it is probably healthier to allow your body to regain control of its own cycles without artificial aids. Having three to four normal cycles before attempting pregnancy would probably be beneficial.

Women who are on the pill for long-term use have been advised to take off three months at a time at two- to four-year intervals. This gives the body a chance to remind itself what a normal cycle is supposed to be. If you want to go off the pill and remain protected, there are other available methods.

The IUD creates a hostile environment in the uterus. With that in mind, the removal of the IUD should also be followed by time off. If scarring and adhesions have not been a problem, a woman should be able to conceive within a three-cycle span. Once again, this allows the body to experience menstrual cycles free from any foreign device, allows it to readjust, and to become ready for pregnancy.

With either the birth control pill or the IUD, cessation means a chance at becoming pregnant. Allowing the body time to readjust means using other means of birth control. Condoms, diaphragms, foams, jellies, sponges, cervical caps, or any combination of these will need to be used. This is vital to maintain control over your choice in timing your conception.

## SUGGESTED READING

*Woman's Body, Woman's Right: A Social History of Birth Control in America*
Linda Gordon
Penguin Books, 1977

*Changing Bodies, Changing Lives*
Ruth Bell
Random House, 1980

*Contraceptive Technology 1982-1983*
Robert Hatcher et al.
Irvington Publishers, 1982

*Birth Control and Controlling Birth*
Helen B. Holmes et al.
Humana Press, 1980

*Women and the Crisis in Sex Hormones*
Barbara Seaman and Gideon Seaman
Bantam Books, 1978

*The Billings Method*
Evelyn Billings, Ann Westmore
Random House, 1980

## RESOURCE GROUPS

Committee for Abortion Rights and Against Sterilization Abuse
17 Murray Street
New York, NY 10007

Reproductive Rights National Network (R2N2)
17 Murray Street
New York, NY 10007

Department of Health and Hospitals
1400 W. 9th Street
Los Angeles, CA 90015
213-260-3151

Ovulation Method Teachers Association
4760 Aldrich Road
Bellingham, WA 98225

National Women's Health Network
224 7th Street, S.E.
Washington, D.C. 20003
202-347-1140

# CHAPTER 15

# DO IT

*"One must not lose desires. They are mighty stimulants to creativeness, to love and to long life."*
—Alexander A. Bogomoletz

## DOWN TO BUSINESS

Not so long ago, your thoughts centered on making changes and choices for a well-prepared life for your child-to-be. You have considered making changes that not only affect you but benefit you for the rest of your life. Choices have been made to improve your health, your wealth, and your security. If the time is right for you, the next step is to go ahead and create a child.

### Where Eggsactly Is Your Ovum?

Just as preconceptional planning is based on timing, so is ovulation. Ovulation is the time between periods when a woman's body is able to conceive. When a baby girl is born, she possesses about 400,000 egg follicles in her ovaries.

When a girl undergoes puberty, her body changes under the influence of hormones leading to secondary sex characteristics. She experiences breast enlargement and pubic and axillary (armpit) hair growth. She begins to menstruate and ovulate, usually around the age of twelve. It is from this point on that pregnancy can and will occur if she has unprotected intercourse.

Hormones fluctuate throughout a woman's monthly cycle. The pituitary gland, deep within the brain, secretes the follicular stimulating hormone (FSH) throughout the first half of the menstrual cycle. This hormone stimulates the development of the eggs in the ovary.

Estrogen and progesterone are secreted by the ovaries. They assist the uterus in preparing for the fertilized egg. The level increases during ovulation, causing physical changes.

As was discussed in chapter 14, there is an increase in cervical mucous and its consistency. There may be a twinge of pain, or a cramp in the lower abdomen, indicating that the egg has ruptured out of the ovary and is ready to be directed toward one of the fallopian tubes.

Once in the tube, the egg lives for 48 hours. If conception does not occur, it is reabsorbed into the body, never to be seen again. If conception does occur, the fertilized egg moves down into the uterus. The uterus is ready for the fertilized egg to be implanted. The lining is thick and rich in nutrients needed by the growing embryo.

If conception does not occur, in about fourteen days the uterine lining is shed in what we know as menstruation. The rule of thumb is that ovulation occurs 14+-2 days before the next period. Whether you are on a 28-day or longer cycle, it should still occur about the same time.

By doing Basal Body Temperature charts and noticing a change in your cervical mucous, you can estimate your ovulation and act accordingly. There are kits available for testing the cervical mucous for pH. The pH tends to increase from the normal during ovulation. These kits are available in drugstores.

It may take a few months of charting to be able to tell exactly when you are ovulating. Once you are sure you know the right time, then make a date for an erotic, hopefully conceptional, encounter. Not everyone can or will want to plan an erotic evening. In fact, a weekend away, a day in bed, or parking just for fun is equally effective. It is important for both partners to be relaxed and rested.

Stress and fatigue decrease sex drives. This can cause some men to be unable to achieve an erection. Our sexuality is influenced by outside wear and tear on our minds. We are all subject to stress, and yet we can manage it by techniques like relaxation, meditation, yoga, and massage.

Timing of conception can be determined with the aid of careful monitoring. What we cannot truly monitor is when and how egg meets sperm. During ovulation, once the egg leaves the ovary, it is brushed into the fallopian tubes by fimbria, or the fringelike structures at the end of the tubes. Once inside the tube, the egg remains in the outer end, awaiting the arrival of the sperm.

Each ejaculation contains about 300 million sperm in 3 to 5 cubic centimeters of semen. The sperm, resembling tadpoles, wiggle their way through the cervix, up through the uterus, and eventually into the tubes.

Sperm can live in the woman's body for two to three days, with some reaching the fallopian tubes in five minutes. Millions make it to the egg, surround it, and begin to attempt fertilization. Only one sperm will break through the surface and ultimately fertilize the egg.

Fertilization includes the dividing of the cells that begin the formation of the baby. This process can take twenty-four hours. By the time your next period is due, the embryo has worked its way down into the uterus and implanted itself in the thick, nutritious uterine lining.

The next eight to ten weeks are a critical time of development for the baby. It is important for the mother to avoid alcohol, drugs, smoking, viruses, and any environmental hazards. With the knowledge that she may be pregnant, the woman should seek prenatal care as soon as possible.

A few ways to enhance fertilization:

- Do not use a lubricant. K-Y jelly can actually destroy sperm. If entry is difficult, use saliva.
- Do not douche or cleanse the vagina after intercourse.
- Use the missionary position (man on top), and remain on your back for about fifteen to twenty minutes.
- After ejaculation has occurred, elevate your hips with a pillow to give the semen extra help in reaching the cervical opening.
- Repeat intercourse a few times. It cannot hurt to add a few more million sperm. It may be necessary to have intercourse for a few days in a row because of the variance in ovulation time.

## MORE THAN A GLOW: YOU ARE PREGNANT

Love making is much more than a way to conceive a child. It is a demonstration of love, an act of pleasure and of comfort. When trying to become pregnant, either or both partners may feel pressured to perform. Working against a clock to get pregnant will make it a more mechanical, regimented act.

It is important to keep in mind that love making should not be turned into a biological battle. You are not considered in need of fertility treatment until you have tried for one year (see chap. 14).

Some couples become so time oriented that if they cannot achieve pregnancy by a certain month and have the baby when they want it, they fall apart. We are not in complete control of our reproductive process. We are only able to learn about our bodies and work with them.

Assuming that your erotic encounter was a success, you are now anxiously awaiting your next period. If your period does arrive right on schedule, you may feel discouraged. It is important to remember that you can and probably will try, try again.

If your period does not show up, you are pregnant and will begin to notice changes in your body. Some obvious signs include the following.

## Breasts

Breast tenderness is a common sign of pregnancy. Touching or bumping your breasts may be uncomfortable. Even now your body begins preparation to nourish your new baby. Continue to wear supportive bras throughout your pregnancy. As breasts grow, the nipple area may become darker in color. This is normal. One of the best things about pregnancy is that you finally develop cleavage.

## Abdomen

By the time you realize you are pregnant, the fetus has already set up house in your uterus. The uterus will begin its growing process. Your abdomen may be tender or feel full. You may even feel the tendency to shield or protect your abdomen from any bumps or bangs. As the belly grows, the skin will stretch and may even feel itchy. Lotions are good for relieving this discomfort.

## Urination

Because the uterus is beginning to grow, it puts pressure on your bladder. You may feel the need to urinate more often. As the uterus grows and rises out of the pelvic cavity, this pressure will be relieved.

Around the fourth month, you may notice a decrease in the need to find the nearest bathroom as soon as possible. You may also notice that you look pregnant and that your clothes fit differently. Do not fight the need to begin wearing maternity clothes. They are made to take pressure off the growing belly and are much more comfortable at this time.

## Nausea and Vomiting

Commonly known as "morning sickness," this symptom of pregnancy is not restricted to mornings alone. It is just that a majority of women tend to be more susceptible to this occurrence in the morning.

Before arising in the morning, try eating saltine crackers. This may help relieve the nausea. Some foods, food smells, or other odors may trigger waves of nausea. This symptom of pregnancy usually passes around the fourth month. Do maintain a nutritious intake of food and fluids for you and your baby.

## Fatigue

The changes your body is experiencing during your pregnancy may leave you feeling tired. It is normal and should be acknowledged. Taking afternoon naps, if possible, will help.

Many women continue working throughout their pregnancy, while some cut back on the number of hours they work. Whatever you decide, be sure to get your rest. Your body is growing a new life. You need rest and tender loving care.

## Emotions

No matter how long a woman has been waiting to become pregnant, her feelings in pregnancy will vary from ambivalence to joy to regrets. Not only is her body changing but her life is changing forever.

The physical changes alone can cause some women anxiety. As if her body is changing almost out of control, she may feel angry. The changes must be viewed as part of a growing process for both her and her baby.

The hormonal changes can lead the pregnant woman to be happy and content one moment and crying the next. It may be a bit of encouragement to know that women tend to become more open with their feelings at this time. Pregnant women may verbalize matters of concern more freely. This is a healthy change that may benefit her for a lifetime.

Emotional ups and downs are normal and should be expected. The pregnant woman realizes the sobering fact that she is changing roles. Her independence will be altered, and her responsibility to this new little person will be great. She may fear how she will perform as a mother, which she understands is a lifetime concern she will have.

Her relationship with her partner may be different. Progressing from wife and lover to mother may be difficult. She views her body as the home for their child while she is pregnant. She may perceive her sexuality as changing.

There are good points about being pregnant and having sex. Some women find sex during pregnancy enjoyable. The increased blood circulation from pregnancy allows for more sensations to be felt. Her larger breasts, once they are no longer sensitive, can also be a source of pleasure for her.

With these emotional changes comes the need for open communication between the woman and her partner. Sharing concerns with your partner will encourage him to share his fears and concerns as well.

The changes of pregnancy, like nausea, vomiting, abdominal tenderness, and breast soreness, will pass in time. By the fourth month or so, these inconveniences will be gone. It is at this time that the baby's first movements may be felt. Quite often, this is a turning point for women. They finally feel like they are pregnant and not just uncomfortable.

## Pregnancy Testing

Once you miss your period and begin to feel "funny," it may be time to have your suspicion of being pregnant confirmed. There are tests that can be done at home. You can purchase them in the drugstore, and all you need to provide is your urine. The kits give specific instructions on how to perform the test. They are fairly accurate and handy. If the test reads positive, then it is time to call your obstetric care giver.

Your obstetrician or midwife may then order a urine test. The test they order is not much different from the one you can perform at home. It is just that some care givers prefer to have a hospital laboratory per form the test, just to be certain. Other care givers will be satisfied with your home test results and suggest you make an appointment for an examination.

The care giver will check your cervix and feel your uterus and may even try to listen for the baby's heartbeat. He will ask you the date of your last period. With this information, the care giver will be able to determine an approximate due date for your baby.

Sometimes if the estimated due date does not seem to correlate with the size of the uterus, the care giver may order a sonogram. This test uses sound waves to create a picture of the inside of the uterus. By seeing the fetus, he can measure its body length and determine its age. A sonogram is a simple procedure done in the X-ray department of a hospital or clinic.

Your doctor or midwife may order a blood test to see how your health is. This test also checks for the Rh factor as well as for rubella immunity. This is a fairly routine test for pregnant women. If there are any problems, the care giver can treat them early in the pregnancy.

You will be asked to return for prenatal checkups every month for several months. The closer to your due date, the more often you will need to be checked.

You will be given prenatal vitamins, which have extra iron. It is important to take these for your health and your baby's. The baby will draw its nourishment from you and deplete you. These vitamins are an extra boost to the healthy diet you have chosen to pursue. At each visit you will be weighed, have your blood pressure checked, and supply a urine sample, preferably the first urine of the day.

As your pregnancy progresses, you will be anxious at times. It is not uncommon for couples to be concerned with their baby's health. No one will be able to reassure you that everything is all right. That will happen when the doctor or midwife places a perfectly healthy little baby in your arms.

The journey from preconceptional woman to pregnant woman has begun. Enjoy your journey, for it is a wonderful fulfilling experience to create and nurture this new life within.

## SUGGESTED READING

*Moving Through Pregnancy*
Elizabeth Bing
Bantam Books, 1975

*Essential Exercises for the Childbearing Year*
Elizabeth Noble
Houghton Mifflin, 1976

*The Complete Book of Pregnancy and Childbirth*
Shelia Kitzinger
Alfred A. Knopf, 1983

*Making Love during Pregnancy*
Elizabeth Bing and Libby Colman
Bantam Books, 1977

*New Life*
Arthur Balaskas and Janet Balaskas
Sidgewick and Jackson, 1983

*What to Expect When You Are Expecting*
Arlene Eisenberg, Heidi Eisenberg Murkoff, Sandee Eisenberg
Hathaway, R.N.
Workman Publishing, 1984

*Pregnancy and Birth*
Tracy Hotchner
Avon Books, 1979

*Your Baby, Your Body*
Carol Dilfer
Crown Publishers, Inc., 1977

*Labor and Birth*
Cecilia Worth
McGraw Hill Book Co., 1983

*Pregnant and Lovin' It*
Lindsay Curtis, M.D., and Yvonne Corales, R.N.
HP Books, 1977

*Pregnancy, Childbirth and the Newborn*
Penny Simkin, R.P.T, Janet Whalley, R.N., B.S.N., Ann Keppler, R.N.
M.N. Meadowbrook, Inc., 1984

## RESOURCE GROUPS

American Foundation for Maternal and Child Health, Inc.
30 Beckman Place
New York, NY 10022
212-759-5510

International Childbirth Education Association
P.O. Box 20048
Minneapolis, MN 55240
612-854-8660

CHAPTER 16

# PREGNANCY AND BIRTH RESPONSIBILITIES
## Onward and Upward

*"I feel the responsibility of the occasion.*
*Responsibility is proportionate to opportunity."*
—Woodrow Wilson

## PREPLANNING MEANS A HEALTHY OUTLOOK

With all the considerations necessary in preconceptional planning, it may seem that pregnancy itself would be the light at the end of the tunnel. Just when you thought all the choices and changes are in place, it becomes apparent that a different type of decision making then takes over.

You have decided to create the best life for yourselves as a couple and potential family. You have worked through life-style changes, financial challenges, and mental and physical health improvements and established a strong foundation for your family-to-be. The responsibility you feel for this child, not yet conceived, is a form of love.

Pregnancy will bring a new focus on what is yet another series of changes and choices. With pregnancy comes a need for some women to feel safe and secure. It is a time of adjustments, both physical and psychological.

It should be understood that there can be a certain amount of vulnerability for the pregnant woman. Never having done this before may create a need for dependency on others. As we know, a pregnant woman is a visual invitation for everyone to give advice. More pregnancy and birth experiences are related by the "experts" to the pregnant woman than ever before. It is a fact that most women remember details of their labors and deliveries, perhaps because it is such a wonderfully memorable experience.

But if a woman has had a bad experience, she tends to relate that quite willingly as well. Being prepared for tales from the front line will allow you to cope at a time when you may feel anxious and even scared about how it will be for you.

Keep in mind that childbirth is not something that just happens to women. You have the opportunity to be either active or passive in your involvement. The International Childbirth Education Association (ICEA) has devised the Pregnant Patient's Bill of Rights, as well as the Pregnant Patient's Responsibilities. The rights statement includes the right to information concerning medication, treatments, and their adverse side effects for the mother and baby. It includes the woman's right to know the names and qualifications of those administering care to her and her baby, as well as the right to access to her baby for care giving, barring any problems. There are numerous other rights that the couple should be aware of. To obtain this knowledge, the couple must realize that they have a responsibility to become self-educated.

The Pregnant Patient's Responsibilities include the responsibility to learn what pregnancy, labor, and birth are all about and to seek a competent care giver and hospital. It is important for the pregnant woman to make arrangements for a support person to accompany her during the labor and delivery.

After birth, parents are responsible for learning about the care of their baby. Other responsibilities include obtaining information regarding the cost of the obstetric care, hospital policies, and how the mother should care for herself during the postpartum period.

It has been proven that the more knowledge a woman has concerning pregnancy, labor, and delivery, the more likely she is to participate in decisions concerning her care. She is also more likely to have a better labor and delivery because she understands what is happening and can work with her body instead of against it. We need to be informed, educated, and responsible as women considering pregnancy and as consumers.

## OBSTETRICIAN, MIDWIFE, OR STORK?

Cartoons used to depict the stork dropping a bundle into the arms of the anxiously waiting couple. If only it were that easy!

With pregnancy comes the need to consult a professional for knowledge and expertise in obstetrics. This means more choices to make concerning who will be the care giver for this important time of life.

### Obstetricians

These physicians have completed additional education in the woman's reproductive and gynecological field. They have surgical training as well. Typically, a pregnant woman is seen by her obstetrician for brief periodic checkups. The checkups include assessing the fetus's position and heartbeat and asking the woman if she is having any problems.

The obstetrician is present when delivery is imminent or if there is a problem requiring close observation. When the delivery is at hand, he is there to assist the birth and make sure everything is progressing normally. He checks the baby briefly for any obvious problems.

During the postpartum period, the obstetrician will check any surgical procedures, such as an episiotomy or cesarean section, that he performed. He answers questions and gives instructions for the mother to follow until he sees her in the office for a six-week checkup.

Obstetricians/gynecologists most often have at least one other partner, sometimes more. The practice may be confusing for a woman who has established a preference for one doctor in particular but who is assisted in labor by another partner. That is the chance taken when employing a physician in a group practice.

Usually these doctors have privileges, or the right to admit and treat patients, at one hospital in particular. This presents a problem if you like the doctor but not the hospital. Seeking a physician who shares your preferences in prenatal care, labor variations, and delivery practices is very important. While it may not seem like the doctor spends a lot of time with the pregnant woman, it is reassuring to know that you are compatible as physician and patient.

## Midwives

Certified nurse midwives (CNM) began practicing in the 1920s. They attended poor women in Appalachia and in New York City. They were concerned about women who could not otherwise afford prenatal care. It was not until 1971 that the American College of Obstetricians and Gynecologists recognized these fine professionals.

They are nurses with experience in obstetrics and gynecology and have additional education in graduate programs. They are specialists in normal pregnancies and birth. If they suspect a woman has complications in her pregnancy or anticipate a problem with the delivery, they readily refer the woman to an obstetrician.

CNMs work with some obstetric practices and hospitals that support their practice. They practice in clinics and alternative birth centers. Midwives are probably best known for their attendance at home births. Midwives are concerned with the woman's entire well-being and encourage women to take control of their prenatal, labor, and delivery responsibilities. They are more actively present during the labor and delivery process.

## EDUCATION IS ESSENTIAL

Whether you employ a midwife or an obstetrician, it is vital to seek early prenatal care. Most care givers will encourage the pregnant couple to attend some type of prenatal classes. Some doctor's offices provide classes taught by their staff. Hospitals quite often offer classes through their maternal-child health division. Still another option is the independent educator who teaches out of their home, church, or other public building.

It is important to seek the educational experience that meets your needs. Some classes offer basic pregnancy knowledge, while others cover breathing, relaxation, and different methods according to the instructor's preference.

When choosing a childbirth class, it is important to research what the class offers in information, the cost, the qualifications of the instructor, and the class size. It is a good idea to shop around for the class that meets your needs.

### Instructor Qualifications

Seventy-five percent of childbirth educators are nurses, with the remainder having backgrounds in physical therapy, education, and related professions. Certification programs for childbirth educators have been established that include workshops, examinations, and labor and delivery observations.

Lamaze is the most popular certification, accounting for 44 percent of certified childbirth educators. ICEA offers certification as well as the Council of Childbirth Educators Association (C/CES) and the American Academy of Husband-Coached Childbirth (AAHC). Some educators have no certification at all.

### Class Size

This is an important area of consideration. A large class, greater than twelve couples, may mean less individual instruction. With a small class, less than six couples, it is difficult to establish the support system of other couples necessary at this time. Location will also influence the comfort of a small or large class. Check into this aspect as well.

## Kinds of Information

The philosophy of the educator and or the hospital will determine what information will be covered. Essential topics include:

• Nutrition
• Exercise and comfort measures
• Life-style changes
• Medications and medical interventions
• Warning signs
• Unexpected outcomes of labor and delivery
• Postpartum adjustments
• Parenting: newborn care and feeding

Ask how much time is spent on these topics as well as breathing and relaxation techniques.

The usual schedule for classes is once a week for six to eight weeks. Each session may be two hours, with a break at midpoint. The typical timing of attending classes is in the last three months of pregnancy, ending a week or two before your due date.

Most classes are held in the evening so that working couples can attend. If you miss a class, ask the instructor if she would be willing to review the material from the previous class. Most instructors would be glad to accommodate these requests.

## Costs

Like everything else, childbirth classes have a price tag. Prices vary depending on the area and whether the classes are affiliated with a hospital or clinic. The average cost is around $45.00. Included in that cost are handouts, usually a handbook, access to a library, viewing of films, a hospital tour, and of course, the educator. It is a worthwhile investment to become educated and be able to make informed decisions concerning your child's birth.

## CHILDBIRTH METHODS

All methods should include the basic understanding that fear and tension cause pain. It is a vicious circle. When you are afraid, you become tense. Tension causes pain to be enhanced, leading to more fear, and so on.

By learning what is happening within your body, you can relax and work with it. The relaxation decreases tension, enabling you to have more control over your labor. Some methods include specific breathing patterns as well.

Our natural tendency is to hold our breath when we are in pain. By holding your breath, you decrease your oxygen supply to your baby and your muscles. The uterus is a muscle that needs oxygen to work efficiently. A contraction is the uterine muscle working.

Between relaxation and breathing you are allowing the uterus to work efficiently. These tools are readily available for any pregnant woman to use in labor.

Different methods place emphasis on certain concepts of labor and delivery.

### Lamaze, or Psychoprophylaxis (PPM) or Mind Prevention

- Encourages active relaxation.
- Teaches conditioned responses to contractions.
- Recommends focusing attention away from the contraction.
- Advocates presence of a support person.

### Dick-Read Method

- Teaches progressive relaxation of the body's muscle groups.
- Teaches breathing techniques that decrease muscle pressure on the uterus.
- Recommends physical exercise to condition body.

### Bradley Method

- Encourages breath control and abdominal breathing.
- Teaches working in harmony with body; general body relaxation.
- Concentrates on minimizing the need for medications.
- Focuses on environmental influences on labor. A dark, quiet atmosphere is considered preferable.

### Home Birth

- Encourages extensive knowledge of labor and delivery.
- Teaches women to trust instincts for giving birth.
- Encourages relaxation.
- Addresses need for actively laboring for a more effective delivery.

It is safe to say that education is a liberating experience for the pregnant couple. Support from your partner includes his participation in these classes. A support person possesses an invaluable wealth of knowledge when the pregnant woman is in the midst of labor.

Support can come in many ways, perhaps best shown by a loving touch and words of encouragement. The pregnant couple should discuss what his concerns may be when it comes to attending the birth. It may be difficult for him to admit his own fears and anxieties. Discussing this area preconceptionally will allow time to learn more about birth and dissolve concerns with knowledge.

## BIG PLANS: BIRTH

With all the other plans you have made, you may want to take the process one step further. Women no longer need to be taken by the hand and led through pregnancy. We are informed and able to make choices right for us, our baby, and our family. Care givers are available for consultation concerning our prenatal health. There is still room available for you to plan the birth of your child.

A birth plan is a written proposal of how you would like your baby's birth to be. It is written with the understanding that your care giver can contribute to it. If you can agree on a plan, then it becomes part of your admission chart. It is then viewed as an order for other staff members to follow.

Should problems arise and medical intervention is needed, the couple must be flexible and work with the health care team. The birth plan is not meant to be a binding contract, inflexible of change for the benefit of either mother or baby.

Some steps to follow when making a birth plan:

- As soon as you are pregnant, find a care giver and hospital willing to work with your decision to create a birth plan.
- Discuss the plan with your care giver, asking for his help. He will be more receptive to this concept.
- Educate yourself. To make a legitimate plan, you must learn all you can about the birth process.
- Use cooperative language in your plan. Acknowledge your willingness to be flexible and use phrases like "if possible" and "our preference would be." Avoid using phrases like "No" or "Do not want."
- Prepare the plan with the possibility of unexpected outcomes. Include an alternate route for such things like cesarean sections, a sick baby, or medical complications for the mother.
- Understand that even if there is a need to take an alternate route, the plan does not have to be abandoned. The staff will help you regain your footing and continue to fulfill your plan if at all possible.

Some options to consider for making your delivery experience personalized include the following:

- Use of personal items for focal points.
- Birthing room with double bed for partner to join the laboring mother.
- Soft, gentle lighting and quiet atmosphere.
- Your personal favorite music.
- Support person present at all times.
- Involvement of partner with birth (cutting cord, delivery of the baby's head and body).
- Personal items for comfort measures. Time alone after birth for partner and baby.

More information on planning this wonderful experience is available. The choices and alternatives are numerous and can be personalized just for you.

## THE GREATEST GIFT

Preconceptional planning is a loving gift from you to your child. By creating changes and making educated choices, you are making her life better, even before she is conceived. When you are secure in your own life, you naturally convey security to your child. This frees both of you to enjoy your life together.

The changes and choices you make will be the right ones for you. As adults we sometimes switch to the role of the child. We seek other adults' approval and allow them to influence our lives. When we doubt our own ability to make choices, we become dependent.

As parents-to-be, you must work together on your choices. Equal input into decision making is important. Your child will be the dependent one in your life. He will rely on your wisdom, common sense, and love for survival. And when he is 20 years old and in a crisis of his own, he may still seek your love and acceptance. Parenting is a lifetime role we play.

Hodding Carter said, "There are only two lasting bequests we can hope to give our children. One of these is roots; the other, wings." By planning for your children, you can give them the roots of a solid foundation and the love to let them fly.

## SUGGESTED READING

*The Birth Primer, A Source Book of Traditional and Alternative Methods
in Labor and Delivery*
Rebecca R. Parfitt
Running Press, 1977

*Having It Your Way*
Vicki Walton
Bantam Books, 1976

*The Rights of the Pregnant Parent*
Valmai Elkins
Waxwing, 1976

*Our Bodies, Ourselves*
The Boston Women's Health Book Collective
Simon and Schuster, 1984

*Planning Your Baby's Birth*
Penny Simkin and Carla Reinke
Pennypress, 1980

*Immaculate Deception: A New Look at Women and Childbirth in America*
Suzanne Arms
Bantam Books, 1977

*Women-Centered Pregnancy and Birth*
Ginny Cassidy-Brinn, Francie Horner, Carol Downer
Cleis Press, 1984

*Childbirth without Fear*
Grantly Dick-Read
Harper & Row, 1978

*Birthrights*
Sally Inch
Pantheon Books, 1984

*The Experience of Childbirth*
Shelia Kitzinger
Penguin Books, 1978

*Changing Childbirth: Family Birth in the Hospital*
Diony Young
Childbirth Graphics, Ltd., 1982

## RESOURCE GROUPS

American Academy of Husband-Coached Childbirth
P.O. Box 5224
Sherman Oaks, CA 91413
818-788-6662

International Childbirth Education Association
P.O. Box 20048
Minneapolis, MN 55420
612-854-8660

ASPO/Lamaze
1840 Wilson Boulevard
Arlington, VA 22201
703-524-7802

Informed Homebirth
P.O. Box 3675
Ann Arbor, MI 48106
313-971-9191

Cesarean Prevention Movement
P.O. Box 152
Syracuse, NY 13210
315-424-1942

National Association of Childbearing Centers
Box 1, Route 1
Perkiomenville, PA 18074
215-234-8068

International Association of Parents and Professionals for Safe
Alternatives in Childbirth (NAPSAC)
P.O. Box 267
Marble Hill, MO 63764
314-238-2010

# GLOSSARY

**Adrenaline:** *A chemical secretion from the adrenal glands, it heightens emotions and is associated with an increase in strength.*

**Allergens:** *Substances that cause an allergic reaction by the body. The immune system responds to allergens, causing reactions.*

**Amniocentesis:** *A procedure performed by a doctor which entails inserting a long, thin needle into the pregnant woman's abdomen. Amniotic fluid is withdrawn for testing purposes.*

**Amoxicillin:** *A semisynthetic penicillin used to treat infections.*

**Anorectic:** *Drug that decreases the appetite.*

**Anticonvulsant:** *Drug that prohibits convulsions from occurring in those prone to them.*

**Arteriosclerosis:** *A chronic disease involving the thickening and hardening of the walls of the arteries. This interferes with blood circulation.*

**Biological clock:** *A mechanism in living organisms by which time-dependent occurrences take place.*

**Calorigenics:** *Drugs that cause an increase in oxygen consumption by the body for the purpose of weight loss.*

**Carbohydrates:** *Those chemical compounds including sugars, starches, and cellulose. These are vital for supplying the body with energy.*

**Cardiac:** *Pertaining to the heart, blood vessels, and circulatory system.*

**Cervix:** *Located at the back of the vagina, it is the opening into the uterus.*

**Cesarean section:** *The delivery of a baby through a surgical incision of the walls of the abdomen and uterus.*

**Clitoris:** *Anterior to the vagina on the genital area, it is the counterpart of the male penis. Stimulation causes sexual excitement and orgasm.*

**Congenital:** *Existing condition before birth. It can be influenced environmentally or by heredity.*

**Cystitis:** *An inflammation of the urinary tract including the bladder.*

**Down's syndrome:** *A chromosomal abnormality also known as Trisomy 21. It is characterized by mental retardation and altered physical appearance.*

**Emphysema:** *A condition of the lungs resulting in air retention in the lungs, which is accompanied by labored breathing.*

**Endocarditis:** *An inflammation of the thin membranes that line the chambers of the heart.*

**Endometriosis:** *A condition in which uterine tissue drifts into the pelvic cavity, causing pain, abnormal bleeding, absence of a period, and possibly infertility.*

**Estrogen:** *Female sex hormone produced by the ovaries and placenta. It is responsible for the development of secondary sex characteristics in females.*

**Fertility:** *The quality of being able to reproduce.*

**Forceps:** *An instrument used to aid in the delivery of the baby's head at the time of birth, if necessary.*

**Genitals:** *The reproductive organs for both men and women.*

**Gestational diabetes:** *A glucose intolerance triggered by the onset of pregnancy. It usually resolves itself after delivery.*

**Gynecologist:** *A doctor who specializes in the study of women's reproductive, urinary, and rectal health.*

**Hormones:** *Chemicals that are secreted by specific organs and increase the function of these organs.*

**Labia:** *The liplike structures of the genital area. They frame either side of the vagina, clitoris, and urethra.*

**Midwife:** *A person who aids a woman in the birth of her child.*

**Nitrate:** *A preservative compound, also found in fertilizers.*

**Nutrients:** *Something that nourishes, especially an ingredient in food.*

**Obstetrician:** *A doctor who specializes in the care of a woman during her prenatal period, labor and delivery, and postpartum recovery.*

**Ovulation:** *The ripening and expulsion of an egg from the ovary. Usually occurring fourteen days prior to the onset of the next period.*

**Paraplegic:** *Someone paralyzed in the lower half of the body.*

**Penicillin:** *A medication derived from mold which is used to treat infections.*

**Perineum:** *The area between the vagina and rectum on women and between the scrotum and rectum on men.*

**pH:** *A measure of acidity or alkalinity of a solution or substance. Normal is 7; higher numbers are alkaline, and lower are acidic.*

**Placenta:** *The vascular, disc-shaped organ connecting the mother and fetus in utero. Nutrients and oxygen are filtered through this life-sustaining organ.*

**Podophyllin solution:** *A solution made from dried Mayapple roots which is used to treat genital warts.*

**Preconceptional:** *The time occurring before the conception of a child.*

**Progesterone:** *A hormone that prepares the uterus for the implantation of a fertilized egg. It is also involved in breast enlargement for nursing and in maintaining a pregnancy.*

**Psychosis:** *A severe mental disorder causing a decrease in normal intellectual and social functioning.*

**Puberty:** *The time in a boy's or girl's life when the reproductive organs mature and become able to produce a child.*

**Rheumatic fever:** *An infectious disease occurring most often in children, resulting in permanent damage to the valves of the heart.*

**Speculum:** *An instrument that is placed in the vagina and gently opened to spread the vaginal walls aside for easier examination of the cervical area.*

**Tetracycline:** *Derived from synthetic compounds, a medication used as an antibiotic for infections.*

**Toxemia:** *Also known as preeclampsia, it is a pregnancy-induced condition resulting in high blood pressure.*

**Tuberculosis:** *A contagious disease that manifests itself in the lungs, bones, and other body parts.*

**Ultrasound:** *This test bounces high frequency sound waves off the fetus, giving an image. The heart as well as the bones and any abnormalities of the baby's structure can be seen. This procedure is also known as a sonogram.*

**Uterus:** *The hollow muscular organ housed deep in the woman's pelvic cavity. It is designed to support the life of a fetus until birth.*

# INDEX

# Other Books from John Muir Publications

## 22 Days Series
These pocket-size itineraries are a refreshing departure from ordinary guidebooks. Each author has an in-depth knowledge of the region covered and offers 22 tested daily itineraries through their favorite destinations. Included are not only "must see" attractions but also little-known villages and hidden "jewels" as well as valuable general information.

**22 Days Around the World** by R. Rapoport and B. Willes (65-31-9)
**22 Days in Alaska** by Pamela Lanier (28-68-0)
**22 Days in the American Southwest** by R. Harris (28-88-5)
**22 Days in Asia** by R. Rapoport and B. Willes (65-17-3)
**22 Days in Australia** by John Gottberg (65-40-8)
**22 Days in California** by Roger Rapoport (28-93-1)
**22 Days in China** by Gaylon Duke and Zenia Victor (28-72-9)
**22 Days in Dixie** by Richard Polese (65-18-1)
**22 Days in Europe** by Rick Steves (65-05-X)
**22 Days in Florida** by Richard Harris (65-27-0)
**22 Days in France** by Rick Steves (65-07-6)
**22 Days in Germany, Austria & Switzerland** by R. Steves (65-39-4)
**22 Days in Great Britain** by Rick Steves (65-38-6)
**22 Days in Hawaii** by Arnold Schuchter (28-92-3)

**22 Days in India** by Anurag Mathur (28-87-7)
**22 Days in Japan** by David Old (28-73-7)
**22 Days in Mexico** by S. Rogers and T. Rosa (65-41-6)
**22 Days in New England** by Anne Wright (28-96-6)
**22 Days in New Zealand** by Arnold Schuchter (28-86-9)
**22 Days in Norway, Denmark & Sweden** by R. Steves (28-83-4)
**22 Days in the Pacific Northwest** by R. Harris (28-97-4)
**22 Days in Spain & Portugal** by Rick Steves (65-06-8)
**22 Days in the West Indies** by C. & S. Morreale (28-74-5)
All 22 Days titles are 128 to 152 pages and $7.95 each, except *22 Days Around the World* and *22 Days in Europe*, which are 192 pages and $9.95.

## "Kidding Around" Travel Guides for Children
Written for kids eight years of age and older. Generously illustrated in two colors with imaginative characters and images. An adventure to read and a treasure to keep.
**Kidding Around Atlanta**, Anne Pedersen (65-35-1) 64 pp. $9.95
**Kidding Around London**, Sarah Lovett (65-24-6) 64 pp. $9.95
**Kidding Around Los Angeles**, Judy Cash (65-34-3) 64 pp. $9.95
**Kidding Around New York City**, Sarah Lovett (65-33-5) 64 pp. $9.95
**Kidding Around San Francisco**, Rosemary Zibart (65-23-8) 64 pp. $9.95

**Kidding Around Washington, D.C.**, Anne Pedersen (65-25-4) 64 pp. $9.95

**Asia Through the Back Door**, Rick Steves and John Gottberg (28-76-1) 336 pp. $15.95

**Buddhist America: Centers, Retreats, Practices**, Don Morreale (28-94-X) 400 pp. $12.95

**Bus Touring: Charter Vacations, U.S.A.**, Stuart Warren (28-95-8) 168 pp. $9.95

**Catholic America: Self-Renewal Centers and Retreats**, Patricia Christian-Meyer (65-20-3) 325 pp. $13.95

**Preconception: A Woman's Guide to Preparing for Pregnancy and Parenthood**, Brenda Aikey-Keller (65-44-0) 236 pp. $14.95

**Complete Guide to Bed & Breakfasts, Inns & Guesthouses**, Pamela Lanier (65-43-2) 512 pp. $15.95

**Elderhostels: The Students' Choice**, Mildred Hyman (65-28-9) 224 pp. $12.95

**Europe 101: History & Art for the Traveler**, Rick Steves and Gene Openshaw (28-78-8) 372 pp. $12.95

**Europe Through the Back Door**, Rick Steves (65-42-4) 432 pp. $16.95

**Floating Vacations: River, Lake, and Ocean Adventures**, Michael White (65-32-7) 256 pp. $17.95

**Gypsying After 40: A Guide to Adventure and Self-Discovery**, Bob Harris (28-71-0) 264 pp. $12.95

**The Heart of Jerusalem**, Arlynn Nellhaus (28-79-6) 312 pp. $12.95

**Indian America: A Traveler's Companion**, Eagle/Walking Turtle (65-29-7) 424 pp. $16.95

**Mona Winks: Self-Guided Tours of Europe's Top Museums**, Rick Steves (28-85-0) 450 pp. $14.95

**The On and Off the Road Cookbook**, Carl Franz (28-27-3) 272 pp. $8.50

**The People's Guide to Mexico**, Carl Franz (28-99-0) 608 pp. $15.95

**The People's Guide to RV Camping in Mexico**, Carl Franz with Steve Rogers (28-91-5) 256 pp. $13.95

**Ranch Vacations: The Complete Guide to Guest and Resort, Fly-Fishing, and Cross-Country Skiing Ranches**, Eugene Kilgore (65-30-0) 392 pp. $18.95

**The Shopper's Guide to Mexico**, Steve Rogers and Tina Rosa (28-90-7) 224 pp. $9.95

**Ski Tech's Guide to Equipment, Skiwear, and Accessories**, edited by Bill Tanler (65-45-9) 144 pp. $11.95

**Ski Tech's Guide to Maintenance and Repair**, edited by Bill Tanler (65-46-7) 144 pp. $11.95

**Traveler's Guide to Asian Culture**, Kevin Chambers (65-14-9) 224 pp. $13.95

**Traveler's Guide to Healing Centers and Retreats in North America**, Martine Rudee and Jonathan Blease (65-15-7) 240 pp. $11.95

**Undiscovered Islands of the Caribbean**, Burl Willes (28-80-X) 216 pp. $14.95

## Automotive Repair Manuals

Each JMP automotive manual gives clear step-by-step instructions together with illustrations that show exactly how each system in the vehicle comes apart and goes back together. They tell everything a novice or experienced mechanic needs to know to perform periodic maintenance, tune-ups, troubleshooting, and repair of the brake, fuel and emission control, electrical, cooling, clutch, transmission, driveline, steering, and suspension systems and even rebuild the engine.

**How to Keep Your VW Alive** (65-12-2) 424 pp. $19.95
**How to Keep Your Rabbit Alive** (28-47-8) 420 pp. $19.95
**How to Keep Your Subaru Alive** (65-11-4) 480 pp. $19.95
**How to Keep Your Toyota Pickup Alive** (28-81-3) 392 pp. $19.95
**How to Keep Your Datsun/ Nissan Alive** (28-65-6) 544 pp. $19.95

## Other Automotive Books

**The Greaseless Guide to Car Care Confidence: Take the Terror Out of Talking to Your Mechanic**, Mary Jackson (65-19-X) 224 pp. $14.95
**Off-Road Emergency Repair & Survival**, James Ristow (65-26-2) 160 pp. $9.95
**Road & Track's Used Car Classics**, edited by Peter Bohr (28-69-9) 272 pp. $12.95

## Ordering Information

If you cannot find our books in your local bookstore, you can order directly from us. Your books will be sent to you via UPS (for U.S. destinations), and you will receive them approximately 10 days from the time that we receive your order. Include $2.75 for the first item ordered and $.50 for each additional item to cover shipping and handling costs. UPS shipments to post office boxes take longer to arrive; if possible, please give us a street address. For air-mail within the U.S., enclose $4.00 per book for shipping and handling. All foreign orders will be shipped surface rate. Please enclose $3.00 for the first item and $1.00 for each additional item. Please inquire for airmail rates.

## Method of Payment

Your order may be paid by check, money order, or credit card. We cannot be responsible for cash sent through the mail. All payments must be made in U.S. dollars drawn on a U.S. bank. Canadian postal money orders in U.S. dollars are also acceptable. For VISA, MasterCard, or American Express orders, include your card number, expiration date, and your signature, or call (505)982-4078. Books ordered on American Express cards can be shipped only to the billing address of the cardholder. Sorry, no C.O.D.'s. Residents of sunny New Mexico, add 5.625% tax to the total.

Address all orders and inquiries to:
John Muir Publications
P.O. Box 613
Santa Fe, NM 87504
(505) 982-4078